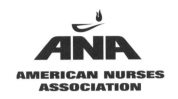

**AMERICAN NURSES
ASSOCIATION**

NURSING INFORMATICS:
SCOPE AND STANDARDS
OF PRACTICE

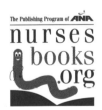

The Publishing Program of ANA

nurses
books
.org

AMERICAN NURSES ASSOCIATION
SILVER SPRING, MARYLAND
2008

Library of Congress Cataloging-in-Publication data

Nursing informatics : scope and standards of practice.
   p. ; cm.
   Includes bibliographical references and index.
   ISBN-13: 978-1-55810-256-9 (pbk.)
   ISBN-10: 1-55810-256-6 (pbk.)
    1. Nursing informatics—Standards. I. American Nursing Association.
   [DNLM: 1. Nursing Informatics—standards. WY 26.5 N9739 2008]

RT50.5N8696 2008
  610.730285—dc22   2007050043

The American Nurses Association (ANA) is a national professional association. This ANA publication— *Nursing Informatics: Scope and Standards of Practice*—reflects the thinking of the nursing profession on various issues and should be reviewed in conjunction with state board of nursing policies and practices. State law, rules, and regulations govern the practice of nursing, while *Nursing Informatics: Scope and Standards of Practice* guides nurses in the application of their professional skills and responsibilities.

Published by Nursesbooks.org
The Publishing Program of ANA

American Nurses Association
8515 Georgia Avenue, Suite 400
Silver Spring, MD 20910-3492
1-800-274-4ANA

The ANA is the only full-service professional organization representing the interests of the nation's 2.9 million registered nurses through its 51 constituent member nurses associations and its 24 specialty nursing and workforce advocacy affiliate organizations that currently connect to ANA as affiliates. The ANA advances the nursing profession by fostering high standards of nursing practice, promoting the rights of nurses in the workplace, projecting a positive and realistic view of nursing, and by lobbying the Congress and regulatory agencies on health care issues affecting nurses and the public.

Design: Scott Bell, Arlington, VA ~ Freedom by Design, Alexandria, VA ~ Stacy Maguire, Sterling, VA ~ *Composition*: House of Equations, Inc., Arden, NC ~ *Editing*: Steven A. Jent, Denton, TX ~ *Proofreading*: Lisa Munsat Anthony, Chapel Hill, NC ~ *Printing*: McArdle Printing, Upper Marlboro, MD

First printing January 2008. Second printing May 2009

ISBN-13: 978-1-55810-256-9   SAN: 851-3481   5M   05/09

ACKNOWLEDGMENTS

Work Group Members (2007)

Nancy Staggers, PhD, RN, FAAN, Chairperson
Michele Calogero, MSN, RN
Margaret F. Budnik, DM, RN
Diane Castelli, RN
Melissa Christensen
Mary F. Clarke, PhD, RN, BC
Tina Dieckhaus, BSN, RN-BC, Leader, Integration and Tenets
Paulette Fraser, MS, RN-BC, Co-leader Metastructures
Josette Jones, PhD, RN-BC, Co-leader Competencies
Sally Kellum, MSN, RN-C
Rosemary Kennedy, MBA, RN, Co-leader NI Standards
Kathleen Krichbaum, RN, PhD
Sheryl LaCoursiere, PhD, RN-BC, Leader, Functional Areas
Angela Lewis, BSN, RN-BC
Teresa McCasky, MBA, BSN, RN-BC
Ramona Nelson, PhD, RN, FAAN, Co-leader, Metastructures
Agnes Padernal, PhD, RN
Amy Peck, RN
Mollie R. Poynton PhD, APRN
Loretta Schlachta-Fairchild, PhD, RN, CHE
Norma Street, MSN, RN
Sharon Sweeney Fee, PhD, RN, Leader, Ethics section
Dawn Weathersby, MS, RN, Co-leader NI Standards
Jill Winters, PhD, RN
Seth Wolpin PhD MPH RN, Co-leader Competencies
Lisa Wynn, MA, RN-BC

ANA Staff

Carol J. Bickford, PhD, RN-BC—Content editor
Yvonne D. Humes, MSA—Project coordinator
Therese Myers, JD—Legal counsel

CONTENTS

THE SCOPE OF NURSING INFORMATICS PRACTICE

Introduction

Nursing informatics (NI) is a specialty that integrates nursing science, computer science, and information science to manage and communicate data, information, knowledge, and wisdom in nursing practice. NI supports consumers, patients, nurses, and other providers in their decision-making in all roles and settings. This support is accomplished through the use of information structures, information processes, and information technology.

The goal of NI is to improve the health of populations, communities, families, and individuals by optimizing information management and communication. These activities include the design and use of informatics solutions and technology to support all areas of nursing, including, but not limited to, the direct provision of care, establishing effective administrative systems, designing useful decision support systems, managing and delivering educational experiences, enhancing lifelong learning, and supporting nursing research (Staggers & Thompson, 2002).

The NI definition remains essentially that found in *Scope and Standards of Nursing Informatics* (2001), but now includes the additional concept of wisdom. The term *individuals* refers to patients, healthcare consumers, and any other recipients of nursing care or informatics solutions. The term *patient* refers to consumers in both a wellness and illness model. The discussion of the definition and goal of nursing informatics evolved from work by Staggers and Thompson (2002).

Nursing informatics is one example of a discipline-specific informatics practice within the broader category of health informatics. NI has become well established within nursing since its recognition as a specialty for registered nurses by the American Nurses Association (ANA) in 1992. It focuses on the representation of nursing data, information, knowledge (Graves & Corcoran, 1989) and wisdom (Nelson & Loos, 1989; Nelson, 2002) as well as the management and communication of nursing information within the broader context of health informatics. Nursing informatics (per Brennan, 2002):

- provides a nursing perspective,
- illuminates nursing values and beliefs,

- denotes a practice base for nurses in nursing informatics,
- produces unique knowledge,
- distinguishes groups of practitioners,
- focuses on the phenomena of interest for nursing, and
- provides needed nursing language and word context to health informatics.

The scope and standards of practice address both informatics nurse specialists (INSs), those formally prepared at the graduate level in informatics or a related field, and informatics nurses (INs), generalists who have experience but are not educated at the graduate level. However, informatics practice is highly complex and in the near future all nurses working in this specialty will have studied at the graduate level.

Nursing Informatics: Scope and Standards of Practice expands on earlier work in NI, builds on historical knowledge (ANA, 1994, 1995, 2001), and includes new, state-of-the-art material for the specialty. Because of rapid changes in related sciences, NI roles, and advances in the science of informatics, a new document was needed. New material in this revision includes: a) the concept of wisdom in NI metastructures, b) redirecting the discussion of roles from job titles to functions that may be integrated into various NI roles and subspecializations, c) identifying commonalities between INSs and other informatics specialists, d) distinguishing between INs and INSs, e) expanding the coverage of NI competencies to describe typical NI competencies for typical NI functional areas, f) expanding the discussion of ethics, human-computer interaction, and the future of NI, g) integrating new functions across clinical practice and NI, and h) changing the section titled "Boundaries of Nursing Informatics" to a discussion of the cross-disciplinary nature of NI that acknowledges the blurred boundaries of other informatics and nursing specialties.

This revised scope and standards document serves in several functions:

- An outline of the attributes and definition of the specialty.
- A reference and guide for educators and NI practitioners.
- A reference for employers and regulatory agencies to assist with developing position descriptions, determining required informatics competencies, and initiating NI positions in health organizations.

- A source document for legal opinions, funding agencies, and others seeking to improve health through nursing informatics.

Metastructures, Concepts, and Tools of Nursing Informatics

To understand NI, first its metastructures, sciences, concepts, and tools should be explained. *Metastructures are overarching concepts used in theory and science.* Also of interest are the sciences underpinning NI, concepts and tools from information science and computer science, human–computer interaction and ergonomics concepts, and the phenomena of nursing.

Metastructures: Data, Information, Knowledge, and Wisdom

In the mid-1980s Blum (1986) introduced the concepts of data, information, and knowledge as a framework for understanding clinical information systems and their impact on health care. He classified the then current clinical information systems according to the three types of objects that these systems processed: data, information, and knowledge. He noted that the classification was artificial, with no clear boundaries, although it did represent a scale of increasing complexity. In 1989, Graves and Corcoran built on these ideas in their seminal study of nursing informatics using the concepts of data, information, and knowledge. They contributed two general principles to NI. The first was a definition of nursing informatics that has been widely accepted in the field. The second contribution of their 1989 contribution was an information model that identified data, information, and knowledge as key components of NI practice (Figure 1).

Drawing from Blum (1986), Graves and Corcoran defined the three concepts as follows:

- Data are discrete entities that are described objectively without interpretation.
- Information is data that are interpreted, organized, or structured.
- Knowledge is information that is synthesized so that relationships are identified and formalized.

Data, which are processed into information and then knowledge, may be obtained from individuals, families, communities, and populations.

Figure 1. Conceptual Framework for the Study of Nursing Knowledge.

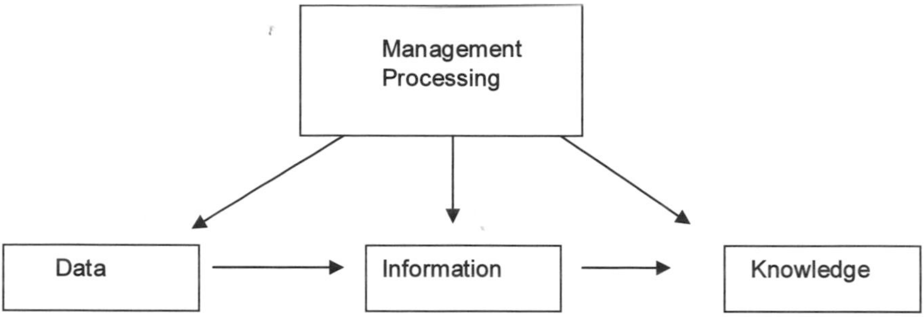

Source: Graves and Corcoran (1989) *Reprinted with permission of the publisher.*

Data, information, and knowledge are of value to nurses in all areas of practice. For example, data derived from direct care of an individual can then be compiled across persons and aggregated for decision-making by nurses, nurse administrators, or other health professionals. Further aggregation can encompass communities and populations. Nurse-educators can create case studies using these data, and nurse-researchers can access aggregated data for systematic study

The vital signs for an individual at a single moment—heart rate, respiration, temperature, and blood pressure—are an example of data. A chronological set of vital signs, placed into a context and used for longitudinal comparisons, is considered information. That is, a dropping blood pressure, increasing heart rate, respiratory rate, and fever in an elderly, catheterized person are recognized as abnormal. The recognition that the person may be septic and therefore may need certain nursing interventions reflects information synthesis (knowledge) based on nursing knowledge and experience.

Figure 2 builds on the work of Graves and Corcoran by depicting the relationship of data, information, knowledge, and a fourth level, wisdom. As data are transformed into information and information into knowledge, each level increases in complexity and requires greater application of human intellect. The X-axis represents interactions within and between the concepts as one moves from data to wisdom; the Y-axis represents the increasing complexity of the concepts and interrelationships.

Figure 2. The Relationship of Data, Information, Knowledge, and Wisdom

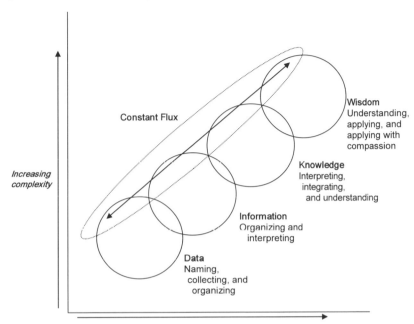

Reprinted with modification from Englebardt & Nelson, 2002, Figure 1-4, page 13 with permission from Elsevier.

Wisdom is defined as the appropriate use of knowledge to manage and solve human problems. It is knowing when and how to apply knowledge to deal with complex problems or specific human needs (Nelson, 1989; Nelson, 2002). While knowledge focuses on what is known, wisdom focuses on the appropriate application of that knowledge. For example, a knowledge base may include several options for managing an anxious family, while wisdom would help decide which option is most appropriate for a specific family. The scope of NI is commensurate with the scope of nursing practice and nursing science, with a concentration on data, information, and knowledge. It is not limited by current technologies. If NI were limited to what a computer can process, the discipline of informatics could not fully appreciate the relationships between nursing science and practice and information science and technology. Nursing informatics must take into consideration how nurses influence technology and how technology influences nursing. Understanding this interaction makes it possible to understand how nurses create knowledge and how they use that knowledge in their practice.

The appropriate use of knowledge involves the integration of empirical, ethical, personal, and aesthetic knowledge into actions. The individual must apply a high level of empirical knowledge in understanding the current situation, apply a professional value system in considering possible actions, be able to predict the potential outcome of these actions with a high level of accuracy, and then have the will power to carry out the selected action in the given environment. An example of applied wisdom integrating these attributes in NI is the appropriate use of information management and technological tools to support effective nursing practice.

The addition of wisdom raises new and important research questions. It challenges the discipline to develop tools and processes for classifying, measuring, and encoding wisdom as it relates to nursing, NI, and informatics education. Research in these directions will help clarify the relationship between wisdom and the intuitive thinking of expert nurses. Such research will be invaluable in building information systems to support expert healthcare practitioners as well as support the less experienced in decision-making.

Two related forces are behind the expansion of the NI model to include wisdom. First, the initial work was limited to the types of objects processed by automated systems in the mid-1980s. However, NI is now concerned with the use of information technology to improve the access and quality of health care that is delivered to individuals, families, and communities. The addition of the concept of wisdom expands the model beyond technology and the processing of objects to include the interaction of the human with the technology and the resultant outcomes.

Second, nurses have been recognized as primary users and processors of information for over 40 years (Jydstrup & Gross, 1966; Zielstroff, 1981). Other authors have focused on the amount of time nurses actually spend administering direct care to patients or the time involved in documentation (Norrie, 1999; Jinks, 2000; Harrison, 2002). In fact, Jydstrup and Gross estimated in the 1960s that nurses in acute care spent 30% to 40% of their time in information processing activities. Hendrickson (1990) determined that nurses spent only 31% of their time with patients. Other aspects of the nursing role included information management with ancillary services.

Sciences Underpinning Nursing Informatics

The work of Graves and Corcoran (1989) was a significant contribution to the NI definition of that was widely accepted in the field in the 1990s— that nursing informatics combines nursing science, information science, and computer science to manage and process nursing data, information, and knowledge to facilitate the delivery of health care. The central notion was that the application of these three core sciences was what made NI unique and differentiated it from other informatics specialties.

Other sciences may be required to solve informatics issues. Turley expanded the model of NI to include cognitive science (1996). Certainly the cognitive aspect of humans is a critical piece for INSs and INs to understand. However, other sciences may be equally critical. If the INS is implementing a system in an institution, for instance, an understanding of organizational theory may be germane (Staggers & Thompson, 2002). As science in general evolves, other sciences may emerge that need to be included in NI models.

Although the core sciences are foundational to the work in NI, the practice of the specialty can be considered an applied science rather than a basic science. The combination creates a unique blend that defines the NI specialty. Further, informatics realizes its full potential in health care when it is grounded in an established discipline; in this case, nursing. Computer and information science will have less impact applied in isolation and outside of a disciplinary framework.

Language as a Tool for Nursing Informatics

Many of the tools used by the informatics nurse and informatics nurse specialist are based on metastructures and concepts that incorporate knowledge from nursing and other health and information sciences. Nursing knowledge is refined by extracting, synthesizing, and analyzing data that defines nursing phenomena. The many different languages and ways of organizing data, information, and knowledge are built on nursing taxonomies and nomenclatures created over decades. ANA (2006a) has formalized these languages and vocabularies (listed in Table 1) after review by the Committee on Nursing Practice Information Infrastructure (CNPII).

Table 1. ANA Recognized Terminologies and Data Element Sets

	Setting Where Developed	Content
Data Element Sets		
NMDS Nursing Minimum Data Set	All Nursing	Clinical Data Elements
NMMDS Nursing Management Minimum Data Set	All Settings	Nursing Administrative Data Elements
*Nursing-Developed Terminologies**		
CCC Clinical Care Classification	All Nursing Care	Diagnoses, Interventions, and Outcomes
ICNP® International Classification of Nursing Practice	All Nursing	Diagnoses, Interventions, and Outcomes
NANDA NANDA International	All Nursing	Diagnoses
NIC Nursing Interventions Classification	All Nursing	Interventions
NOC Nursing Outcomes Classification	All Nursing	Outcomes
Omaha System Omaha System	Home Care, Public Health, and Community	Diagnoses, Interventions, and Outcomes
PCDS Patient Care Data Set* (retired)	Acute Care	Diagnoses, Interventions, and Outcomes
10. PNDS Perioperative Nursing Data Set	Perioperative	Diagnoses, Interventions and Outcomes
Multidisciplinary Terminologies		
ABC ABC Codes	Nursing and Other	Interventions
LOINC® Logical Observation Identifiers, Names, and Codes	Nursing and Other	Outcomes and Assessments
SNOMED CT Systematic Nomenclature of Medicine Clinical Terms	Nursing and Other	Diagnoses, Interventions, and Outcomes

Source: ANA 2006a. (* Except for the retired PCDS, all nursing-developed terminologies are still currently in use.)

To promote the integration of standardized terminologies into information technology solutions, ANA's Nursing Information and Data Set Evaluation Center (NIDSEC) develops and disseminates standards pertaining to information systems that support the documentation of nursing practice, and evaluates voluntarily submitted information systems against these standards.

At a higher level of structure, several resources facilitate interoperability between different systems of concepts and nomenclature. For instance, the Systematized Nomenclature of Medicine, or SNOMED CT (IHTSDO, 2007), is considered a universal healthcare reference terminology and messaging structure. SNOMED CT enables one nursing terminology system to be mapped to another, e.g., Omaha System with North American Nursing Diagnosis Association (NANDA), Nursing Interventions Classification (NIC), and Nursing Outcomes Classification (NOC). On a larger scale, the Unified Medical Language System (UMLS) of the National Library of Medicine (NLM, 2006) incorporates the work of over one hundred vocabularies, including SNOMED CT. The informatics nurse and informatics nurse specialist must be aware of these tools, and may be called upon to understand the concepts of one or more languages, the relationships between concepts, and integration into existing vocabularies for a given organization.

The importance of languages and vocabularies cannot be overstated. Informatics nurses must seek a broader picture of the implications of their work, and the uses and outcomes of languages and vocabularies for end users. For instance, nurses mapping a home care vocabulary to an intervention vocabulary must see beyond the technical aspect of the work. They must understand that a case manager for a multi-system health organization or a home care agency may be basing knowledge of nursing acuity and case mix on the differing vocabularies that they have integrated. The INS must attempt to envision the varied uses of the data, information, and knowledge that have been created.

Concepts and Tools from Information Science and Computer Science

Tools and methods from computer and information sciences are fundamental to NI, including:

- Information technology
- Information structures

- Information management

- Information communication

Information technology includes computer hardware, software, communication, and network technologies, derived primarily from computer science. The other three elements are derived primarily from information science. Information structures organize data, information, and knowledge for processing by computers. Information management is an elemental process by which one files, stores, and manipulates data for various uses. Information communication enables systems to send data and to present information in a format that improves understanding. The use of information technology distinguishes informatics from more traditional methods of information management.

Human–Computer Interaction and Related Concepts

Human–computer interaction (HCI), usability, and ergonomics are concepts of fundamental interest to the INS. Essentially, HCI deals with people, software applications, computer technology, and the ways they influence each other (Dix, Finlay, Abowd, & Beale, 2004). Elements of HCI are rooted in psychology, social psychology, and cognitive science. However, the design, development, implementation, and evaluation of applications derive from applied work in computer science, a specific discipline (in this case nursing), and information science. For example, an INS would assess a medication ordering application before purchase to determine whether the design complements the way nurses cognitively process orders.

A related concept is usability, which deals with human performance during computer interactions for specific tasks in a specific context. Usability means the efficiency and effectiveness of an application. An INS might study the ease of learning an application, the ease of using it, the speed of task completion, or errors that occur during use when determining which system or application would best fit a nursing unit.

In the United States, the term ergonomics typically is used to describe the design and implementation of equipment, tools, and machines related to human safety, comfort, and convenience. Commonly, the term ergonomics refers to attributes of physical equipment or to principles of arrangement of equipment in the work environment. For instance, an INS may have a role in ensuring that sound ergonomics principles are used in an intensive care unit to select and arrange various devices to support workflow for cross-disciplinary providers as well as patients' families.

HCI, usability, and ergonomics are typically subsumed under the rubric of human factors, or how humans and technology relate to each other. The overall goal is to design software, devices, and equipment to promote optimal task completion. Optimal task completion includes the concepts of efficiency and effectiveness; it also considers the safety of the user. The INS and IN must understand all these concepts to successfully develop, select, implement, and evaluate information structures and informatics solutions.

The importance of human factors in healthcare was elevated with the Institute of Medicine's 2001 report. Before this, HCI and usability assessments and methods were being incorporated into health at a glacial speed. In the past five years the number of HCI and usability publications in healthcare has increased substantially. Vendors have installed usability laboratories and incorporated usability testing of their products into their systems life cycles. The FDA has mandated usability testing as part of their approval process for new devices (FDA, 2007a). Thus, HCI and usability are critical concepts for INs and INSs to understand. Numerous usability methods and tools are available, e.g., heuristics (rules of thumb), naturalistic observation, and think-aloud protocols.

Phenomena of Nursing

The metaparadigm of nursing comprises four key concepts: nurse, person, health, and environment. Nurses make decisions about interventions from their unique perspectives. Nursing actions are based upon the inter-relationships between the concepts and are related to the values nurses hold relative to them. Decision-making is the process of choosing among alternatives. The decisions that nurses make can be characterized by both the quality of decisions and the impact of the actions resulting from those decisions. As knowledge workers, nurses make numerous decisions that affect the life and well-being of individuals, families, and communities. The process of decision-making in nursing is guided by the concept of critical thinking. "Critical thinking is the intellectually disciplined process of actively and skillfully using knowledge to conceptualize, apply, analyze, synthesize, and/or evaluate data and information as a guide to belief and action." (Scriven & Paul, 2003)

Clinical wisdom is the ability of the nurse to add experience and intuition to a situation involving the care of a person (Benner, Hooper-Kyriakidis, & Stannard, 1999). Wisdom in informatics is the ability of the informatics nurse specialist to evaluate the documentation drawn from a health information system (HIS) and the ability to adapt or change the system settings or parameters to improve the workflow of the clinical nurse.

Nurses' decision-making can be described as an array of choices that include specific behaviors, as well as cognitive processing of one or more issues. For example, nurses use data transformed into information to determine interventions for persons, families, and communities. Nurses make decisions about potential problems presented by an individual and about recommendations to address those problems. They also make decisions in collaboration with other healthcare professionals such as physicians, pharmacists, or social workers. Decisions also may occur outside the practice environment, as in executive offices, classrooms, and research laboratories.

An information system collects and processes data and information. Decision support systems are computer applications designed to facilitate human decision-making. Decision support systems are typically rule-based: they use a knowledge base and a set of rules to analyze data and information and provide recommendations. Other decision support systems are based on knowledge models induced directly from data, regression, or classification models that predict characteristics or outcomes.

An expert system is a decision support system that implements the knowledge of human experts. Recommendations take the form of alerts, such as calling user attention to abnormal lab results or potential adverse drug events, or suggestions, e.g., appropriate medications, therapies, or other actions (Haug, Gardner, & Evans, 1999). Whereas control systems implement decisions without involvement of a user, decision support systems merely provide recommendations and rely on the wisdom of the user to apply them. As Blum (1986) demonstrated, the concepts of data, information, knowledge, and wisdom exemplify different levels of automated systems. The relationships between these concepts and information, decision support, and expert systems are represented in Figure 3.

Figure 3. Levels and Types of Automated Systems

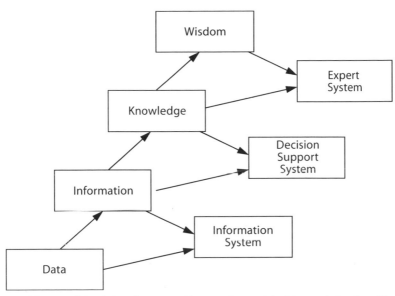

Reprinted from Englebardt & Nelson, 2002, Figure 1-5, page 14 with permission from Elsevier.

In summary, the INS must navigate the complex relationships between the following elements and understand how they facilitate decision-making:

- Data, information, knowledge, and wisdom
- Nursing science, information science, computer science, cognitive science and other sciences of interest
- Nurse, person, health, and environment
- Information structures, information technology, management and communication of information

References: Introduction, Metastructures, Concepts, and Tools

American Nurses Association (ANA). (2006a). *ANA Recognized Terminologies and Data Element Sets*. Retrieved October 10, 2007 from http://nursingworld.org/npii/terminologies.htm

Benner, P.E., Hooper-Kyriakidis, P.L., & Stannard, D. (1999). *Clinical wisdom and interventions in critical care: A thinking-in-action approach.* Philadelphia: W.B. Saunders.

Bellinger, G., Castro, D., & Mills, A. (2004). Data, information, knowledge, and wisdom. Retrieved October 10, 2007 from http://www.systems-thinking.org/dikw/dikw.htm

Blum, B. (1986). *Clinical information systems.* New York: Springer-Verlag.

Clark, D. (2004) The continuum of understanding. From *The way of systems.* Retrieved October 10, 2007 from http://www.nwlink.com/~donclark/performance/understanding.html.

Dix, A., Finlay, J., Abowd, G., & Beale, R. (2004). *Human-computer interaction.* Harlow, England: Pearson, Prentice Hall.

Englebardt, S. & Nelson, R. (2002) *Health care informatics: An interdisciplinary approach.* St. Louis: Mosby-Year Book, Inc.

Graves, J., & Corcoran, S. (1989). The study of nursing informatics. *Image, 21*(4), 227–230.

Harrison, L. (2002). Nursing activity in general intensive care. *Journal of Clinical Nursing, 11*(2), 158–67.

Haug, P., Gardner, R., & Evans, S. (1999). Hospital-based decision support. In E.S. Berner (Ed.), Clinical *Decision Support Systems: Theory and Practice*, pp. 77–104. New York: Springer-Verlag.

Hendrickson, G. (1990). How do nurses use their time? *Journal of Nursing Administration, 20*(3), 31–38.

Institute of Medicine (IOM). (2001). *Crossing the quality chasm: A new health system for the 21st century.* Washington, DC: National Academies Press.

International Health Terminology Standards Development Organization (IHTSDO). (2007). *SNOMED-CT.* Retrieved October 10, 2007 from http://www.ihtsdo.org/.

Jinks, A.M. (2000) What do nurses do? An observational survey of the activities of nurses on acute surgical and rehabilitative wards. *Journal of Nursing Management* 8(5), 273–279.

Jydstrup, R.A., & J.J.Gross. (1966) Cost of information handling in hospitals. *Health Services Research* 1(3): 235–271.

Nelson, R. (2002). A placeholder for a missing ref item for a citation in this section. *Nursing Miscellany: A Catch-all Journal of the Fourth Kind,* 42(4), 656–666.

Nelson, R., & Joos, I. (1989). On language in nursing: From data to wisdom. *PLN Vision.* p. 6.

Norrie, P. (1997). Nurses' time management in intensive care. *Nursing Critical Care,* 2(3), 121–125.

Norrie, P. (1999) The parameters that cardiothoracic intensive care nurses use to assess the progress or deterioration of their patients. *Nursing Critical Care,* 4(3), 133–137.

Scriven, M., & Paul, R. (2003). Defining critical thinking. Santa Rosa, CA.: Foundation for Critical Thinking. Retrieved December 13, 2007 from http://www.criticalthinking.org

Staggers, N., & Thompson, C.B. (2002). The evolution of definitions for nursing informatics: A critical analysis and revised definition. *Journal of the American Medical Informatics Association,* 33(1), 75–81.

Turley, J.P. (1996). Toward a model for nursing informatics. *Image: Journal of Nursing Scholarship,* 28(4), 309–313.

Zielstroff, Z. Z. (1981). Yet another placeholder for a missing ref item for a citation in this section. *Nursing Miscellany: A Catch-all Journal of the Fourth Kind,* 42(4), 666–669.

Functional Areas for Nursing Informatics

Two recent studies illuminate the current work of INs. Newbold (personal communication, January 17, 2006) created a database of job titles for nurses working in informatics beginning in the early 1980s. As of early 2006, the database included titles for 6338 members of nursing and informatics organizations, conference attendees and participants on NI electronic discussion lists. However, the top 50 job titles did not consistently map to their responsibilities and activities. INs with different titles may actually be performing the same functions, and INs with the same titles may perform very different functions.

A 2007 Health Information Management and Systems Society (HIMSS) survey of 776 informatics nurses categorized NI work into job responsibilities as opposed to job titles (HIMSS, 2007). The top job responsibility of respondents was systems implementation (45%), down from 67% in 2004. The second and third top job responsibilities reported by HIMSS respondents were system development (41%) and liaison (35%).

Not only are there assorted titles and activities within nursing informatics, the environments in which INSs and INs practice are many and evolving. Initially, NI focused nearly exclusively on the hospital setting. Now INs work in such diverse settings as home health and hospice agencies, nursing homes, public and community health agencies, physician offices, and ambulatory care centers. They are employed by medical device vendors, large and small software companies, web content providers, disease management companies, and government agencies, in numerous settings (Sensmeier, West, & Horowicz, 2004). Across environments , INSs and INs commonly practice in interdisciplinary healthcare environments and are often expected to interact with information technology (IT) professionals during all phases of the systems life cycle. And more commonly than in the past, INs may be the IT professionals themselves.

Nursing informatics supports multiple constituencies and stakeholders such as cross-disciplinary team members, healthcare consumers, information technology professionals, and healthcare agencies and organizations. INSs are particularly well suited to work in multidisciplinary and interdisciplinary environments. After all, nurses have planned, implemented, and coordinated activities involving multiple constituencies in a consumer-centered fashion from their earliest days.

INSs use scientific and informatics principles. More importantly, they employ creative strategies in meaningful informatics solutions. INSs also bring unique perspectives of cross-disciplinary work, solid understanding of operational processes, and the value of consumer advocacy to informatics functions. INs and INSs may find that they need varying kinds of advanced preparation to match the informatics project at hand. For instance, an INS coordinating the implementation of a learning management system may benefit from advanced preparation in adult education.

Many registered nurses have worked on informatics initiatives for many years and have built their knowledge base and expertise from on-the-job experience. The evolving mandate for electronic information systems and the increasing complexity of healthcare services and practice have raised the bar for the nursing professional. Select informatics competencies will soon be required in all undergraduate and graduate nursing curricula. Accredited graduate level educational programs for this specialty nursing practice were first offered in 1989 and are now more widely available, especially through distance education and online programs. Rather than offer discipline-specific informatics programs, some universities have elected to embrace an interdisciplinary approach and offer graduate studies in health informatics or bioinformatics. A graduate level informatics degree is becoming the standard.

Professional certification as an informatics nurse became a reality in late 1995 when the American Nurses Credentialing Center (ANCC) offered the nursing informatics certification exam as its first computer-based examination. Informatics nurses and informatics nurse specialists may elect to pursue other pertinent certifications in areas such as project management, security and privacy, network management, and knowledge management. Employers are beginning to use certification as a preferred characteristic during the hiring process.

Because of the tendency to confuse roles with titles and the vast number of position titles and lack of standardization among them, this section describes the *functional areas* for INSs and INs. The following present overall functional areas of nursing informatics:

- Administration, leadership, and management
- Analysis
- Compliance and integrity management

- Consultation

- Coordination, facilitation, and integration

- Development

- Educational and professional development

- Policy development and advocacy

- Research and evaluation

The last discussion in this section describes integrated functions, especially those crossing clinical practice and informatics. INSs may be in positions that focus primarily in one functional area, or, more frequently, several functional areas are combined within a particular NI position.

Administration, Leadership, and Management

As is true of administration in general, leadership and management functions in nursing informatics consist of both higher-level and mid-level administrative functions (ANA, 2004b). Increasingly, INSs are attaining senior leadership positions. Positions may be titled President, Director, Chief Information Officer (CIO), or similar leadership titles (AMIA, 2006a; Staggers & Lasome, 2005; Greene, 2004). In this functional capacity, nursing informatics leaders are expected to be visionary and establish the direction of large-scale informatics solutions. The nursing informatics leader often serves as a catalyst for developing strategic plans, creating national or system policies and procedures, and serving as champion for complex projects and disparate system users.

In mid-level management, INSs may supervise resources and activities for all phases of the systems life cycle. These activities may include needs analysis, requirements gathering, design, development, selection and purchase, testing, implementation, and evaluation of systems to support all facets of nursing and healthcare delivery. In all levels, leadership combines the skills of superb communication, change management, risk assessment, and coalition building with political finesse, business acumen, and strategic application knowledge.

INSs serving in this functional area may put most of their energy into leadership and management. In other positions, administration may be part of a position merged with other functional areas. Examples might include:

- INS at a large hospital system, supervising an implementation and education team, representing nursing interests on various IT committees, performing project management for multiple documentation projects, and having oversight of nursing standards and vocabularies used in applications.

- Project director for a clinical software company, managing implementation teams for various client projects (hospitals to ambulatory facilities) and consulting with clients on all aspects of systems selection, customization, adoption, and use of software.

- Grants administrator for an information science research agency seeking and writing grants that would fund NI-related projects, designing budgets, and ensuring optimal allocation of resources.

Analysis

Data can be aggregated and analyzed in an infinite number of ways to synthesize knowledge, inform decision support and outcomes management, and advance the science of nursing informatics. The INS may use a number of tools to accomplish these ends. Taxonomies and clinical vocabularies can be used to tag consumer data for higher-level analysis. Meta-analysis can identify large-scale trends across multiple groups of data. Systems and requirements analysis can track the flow of data in a system, customized to end-user needs. Workflow analysis can detail steps taken for a number of tasks.

A major responsibility of the INS is to understand work process flows, the particular informatics solution, and how these affect each other. Processes must be designed for successful interactions between users and computers. Competency in formal systems analysis techniques and use of statistical software may be required. These techniques compare the capabilities and limitations of systems to be installed, and where changes must be designed. Discrepancies between the current and ideal systems must be identified and redundancies removed. The clinical analysis process also may include tools and systematic methods, such as process redesign, to enhance safety and reduce inefficiencies.

INSs may also engage in the process of knowledge discovery in databases (KDD). Using sound methodologies and practical evidence-based recommendations, the INS can discover information and knowledge related to diverse areas of nursing practice. Knowledge discovery methods, including data mining and machine learning methods, can be applied along with statistical analysis and data visualization techniques, to identify and understand patterns in very large data stores, such as enterprise data warehouses (Fayyad, 1996).

Analysis is also required with languages and taxonomies. Nursing languages such as Nursing Interventions Classification (NIC), Nursing Outcomes Classification (NOC), and medical vocabularies must be periodically re-evaluated for their applicability and currency (CNCCE, 2004). Analysis of a meta-database such as the Unified Medical Language System or UMLS (NLM, 2006) requires knowledge of nursing as well as medical vocabularies in order to analyze groups of taxonomies, a task ideally suited to the expertise of an INS.

Analysis of outcomes may be related to any domain of nursing practice—clinical, education, research, or administration. The complexity and levels of outcomes must be determined for healthcare consumers, populations, and institutions. Analysis can include the use of Human-Computer Interaction (HCI) principles and methods. In that domain, INSs use HCI tools and methods such as heuristics and cognitive walk-through to analyze the fit of users, tasks, and contexts. Other tools are also available. Analysts use system tools to maintain data integrity and reliability, facilitate data aggregation and analysis, identify outcomes, and develop performance measurements. These techniques allow nurses to contribute to building a knowledge base consisting of the data, information, theories, and models used by nurses and other stakeholders in decision-making and support of healthcare. Analysis activities may include:

- A nursing analyst in a hospice setting tracks health consumer data to establish a weighted case mix to determine nursing personnel allocations.

- A quality improvement (QI) specialist in a hospital system aggregates multi-site research data related to diagnosis and nursing procedures.

- A quality assurance (QA) analyst works with nurse managers to re-tool current work processes after examining existing system data in customized QA reports.

- An analyst applies knowledge discovery methods to warehoused electronic data to build a predictive model of patient falls.

Compliance and Integrity Management

With the advent of national laws advocating for the protection of health information, INSs are responsible for ensuring the ethical use of data, as well as data integrity, security, and confidentiality of protected health information. One function of the INS is knowledge and application of ethical standards. The Health Insurance Portability and Accountability Act (HIPAA) of 1996 has obliged healthcare organizations to revise operational procedures for staff, as well as technical processes, to maintain compliance. INSs must be fluent in these new requirements; they are involved in creating, implementing, and assuring organizational change to meet new legislative mandates. Compliance also includes adherence to national and international standards. These standards may include those from government agencies, such as the Food and Drug Administration (FDA) and National Institutes of Health (NIH), as well as accreditation organizations such as the Joint Commission.

Ethical issues related to consumer privacy abound. One arises from knowledge discovery in databases (KDD), where prediction of outcomes based on individual characteristics, behavior, or usage may be used to stratify groups of people. Although used in a variety of industries, KDD remains controversial in health care. Adequate HIPAA protections must be in place, and relevant ethical issues must be considered in all phases of data retrieval and analysis. For example, analysis of genomic data may result in sensitive predictions of susceptibility to disease. Given the explosive growth of large data stores and enterprise data warehouses, KDD is important for extraction of useful information and knowledge; nevertheless, protecting consumer privacy is vital. The INS can help ensure a balance between access and privacy.

The emerging sciences of genomics and bioinformatics could be used to predict risk for certain diseases, and thus insurability risk. Ethical issues surround the use of new products, such as embedded technologies and radio-frequency identification (RFID) and their application in caring for persons with Alzheimer's disease and other dementias. As the profession matures, some of these issues will be resolved and standards will be established. Requirements will continue to evolve; see the section, Future of NI, on page 61. Examples of compliance and integrity management activities include:

- The security officer for a hospital ensures that HIPAA standards are met by software vendors within the organization, periodically monitors software audit logs for breaches, and ensures that passwords are not shared and backup and disaster procedures are in place and operational.

- A compliance officer for a state health agency writes and enforces policies that conform to state and national laws respecting records retention.

- A care coordinator administrator for a hospital system ensures the confidentiality of data transmitted via telehealth and telemedicine devices

Consultation

Informatics nurses and informatics nurse specialists apply informatics knowledge and skills to serve as a resource to clients, both formally and informally, in external and internal settings. Consultants are experts in the areas of process redesign, strategic IT planning, system implementation, writing informatics publications, evaluating clinical software products, working with clients to write requests for proposals, performing market research, and assisting in the planning of conferences, academic courses, and professional development programs. These expert INSs may work for a consulting firm, be employed as staff of the organization where they consult, own an independent practice, or be recognized as an expert by writing about NI and speaking at NI-related events. Flexibility, good communication skills, breadth and depth of clinical and informatics knowledge, and excellent interpersonal skills are needed to respond to rapidly changing projects and demands. Examples include:

- Consulting with individuals and groups in defining healthcare information problems and identifying methods for implementing, utilizing, and modifying IT solutions and data structures to support healthcare access, delivery, and evaluation.

- Consulting as the project manager, ensuring that team members are performing duties as assigned and the project is completed within budget.

- Consulting with clients in writing requests for proposals to elicit vendor bids for informatics solutions and in evaluating vendor responses.

Coordination, Facilitation, and Integration

One of the most common NI roles is implementing informatics solutions. Nurses are particularly well suited for IT implementation, as it essentially follows the nursing process of assessment, planning, implementation, and evaluation (ANA, 2004a). Also, the INS frequently serves as a bridge between informatics solution users and IT experts. The IN or INS serves as project coordinator, facilitating change management and integrating the information and technology to transform processes. In this role, project management knowledge and skills are essential to the successful outcome of the project. Project coordination can range from small, department-centered applications to enterprise-wide electronic health record (EHR) installations, from coordinating a rehabilitation module in the rehabilitation unit to installing a complete EHR in 42 hospitals.

Of particular note, effective communication is an inherent part of many NI functions, but especially related to coordination, facilitation, and integration. The IN and INS are at the hub of cross-disciplinary communication among professional disciplines and IT, serving as translators and integrators for system requirements and impacts.

In another instance, informatics nurses serve as the liaison between software engineers and end users. In this capacity, the informatics nurse ensures that the necessary testing or research is performed to determine the end user's needs, and that this information is conveyed to the software engineers in terms they can understand. Once the engineer has created a product, the INS evaluates the utility of the product from the viewpoint of the end user. This liaison type of facilitation and coordination occurs in multiple environments. Ensuring the integration of nursing vocabularies and standardized nomenclatures in applications is another example. In this case INSs also act as usability experts and recommend ideal formats for the utilization of technology. Examples of coordination, facilitation, and integration might include:

- The project coordinator for a statewide electronic medical record implementation coordinates all aspects of the project and supervises a cross-disciplinary team to train public health personnel to use the application.

- The project manager for a clinical software company manages the resources and activities using tools such as project management software and project plans for clients whose responsibilities cross inpatient and ambulatory areas

- The clinical liaison for a telehealth software vendor communicates with providers and consumers to ensure that all parties are agreeable to development and implementation plans, and ensures that providers using the system receive adequate technical education.

- A usability expert on a software development team advises software engineers on screen design from the standpoint of clinical documentation needs, performs or coordinates testing of iterative designs, and validates clinical requirements with the users.

Development

Development was listed as the second most common responsibility of HIMSS NI respondents in 2007 (HIMSS, 2007). A developer is responsible for translating user requirements into effective informatics solutions. INSs are involved in a vast array of development activities, from conceptualizing models for applications, to software and hardware design, to the design of education manuals, to the design of complex technology networks. As part of this function, INSs and INs participate in the process of design, iterative development, testing, and dissemination of quality informatics solutions for nurses, interdisciplinary providers, and consumers. An understanding of the information needs of nurses and the nursing profession, consumers and consumer care processes, as well as knowledge of business, client services, projected market directions, product design, product development methods, market research, contemporary programming, systems design, and modeling language are essential for practicing in a development environment.

Adherence to national standards and regulatory requirements is also essential to any development work. In order to ensure interoperability between systems, INSs and INs involved in system development must be knowledgeable about international standards requirements. Existing standards include Health Level Seven (HL-7), International Organization for Standardization (ISO), Current Procedural Terminology (CPT), International Classification of Disease (ICD), and Digital Image Communication (DICOM) group standards, as well as Section 508 accessibility standards (Hammond, 1995; GSA, 2006). An understanding of the current work on standards is mandatory. Development responsibilities might include:

- A developer with a personal health record software vendor creates user-friendly screens for consumers to enter information as well as screens for nurses to display and interpret the data.

- A database administrator with a large multi-site teaching organization manages an expanded nursing vocabulary set for inpatient, ambulatory, and home health nursing documentation.

- A nurse web content developer for a consortium creates and validates content for educational handouts, help and tool tips for user interfaces that display national guidelines, and educational tools. This would include new and innovative tools for knowledge dissemination.

- A programmer in a hospital IT department codes software for documenting diabetic education.

Education and Professional Development

Education is a critical component of many NI functions and may directly affect the success or failure of any new or modified IT solution. Vendors of information systems frequently use the term *training* when referring to client education. In nursing, however, the broader label of *education* is used. Adherence to solid educational principles is a component of education and professional development (ANA, 2000). Teaching nurses and nursing students, healthcare consumers, and other interdisciplinary health team members about the effective and ethical uses of information technology, as well as NI concepts and theories, is essential for the optimal use of informatics solutions in nursing practice. Ever-changing requirements in health information technology make continuing education essential as well. INSs and INs in this capacity develop, implement, and evaluate educational curricula and educational technologies that meet the needs of students.

In this role, educators and trainers assess and evaluate informatics skills and competencies while providing feedback to students regarding the effectiveness of the learning activity and the students' ability to demonstrate newly acquired skills. Educators and trainers manage, evaluate, report, and utilize data and information related to students and the educational delivery system. These INSs are innovators in defining and developing educational technologies, integrating the solutions into the educational and practice environments, and challenging organizations to consider and adopt innovative informatics solutions.

The INS must consider information competency as well as literacy. Computer literacy is a core competency needed in health care, and should be taught in nursing curricula at all levels. In addition, information literacy must be integrated into practice and used to support knowledge management. These are the foundations of informatics competencies.

Education and professional development includes not only INSs, INs, and end users, but also consumers. With the advent of distance technologies such as telehealth and Internet-based consumer-accessible applications, new competencies are needed to ensure that health information is displayed to consumers at an appropriate level of understanding; support staff may not be available in person. Cultural issues, language considerations, and literacy of consumers may not be apparent, and materials may need to be more fully assessed for appropriate presentation and understanding.

INSs may need to ensure presentation of content for web-based knowledge portals of private and government health organizations that may exist in multiple locations, or only virtually. Health information may need to be distilled for consumer consumption. Thus education and professional development involve not only educating INs and INSs, but also developing appropriate interfaces for the consumer. Education and professional development might include:

- A professor of nursing at a major university teaches graduate nursing students enrolled in a nursing informatics degree program or teaches nursing students at all levels the basic NI principles and foundations.

- A clinical preceptor for newly hired nurses and students provides orientation about telehealth, engages them in using telehealth technology, and role models the telehealth nurse responsibilities of monitoring physiologic parameters and providing consumer education.

- An educator for a vendor travels internationally to train nurses on the product's operations, capabilities, troubleshooting, limitations, and benefits.

- A staff development liaison for a large hospital educates nurses and other end users about how to integrate clinical applications into their work processes.

- A help desk team member for a large oncology center works with users as product upgrades are released, answers clinical user questions on the phone or in person, and trouble-shoots user problems.

- A patient education coordinator facilitates electronic consumer health resources.

- A web developer is responsible for development, maintenance, and presentation of disease content for a hospital web portal.

Policy Development and Advocacy

INSs play a key role in formulation of health policy, particularly bringing expertise in data and information content, data structures, and IT solutions with those attributes. Policy development may be at any level—international, national, state, professional specialty, institution or a work unit. INSs are experts in defining the data needed and the structure, management, and availability of those data for decision-making. As such, they advocate for consumers, providers, and the enterprise, and articulate relevant issues from a nursing perspective. Policy-related activities may include developing, writing, implementing, and evaluating guidance. Regardless of the level or activity, INSs are partners in setting health policy, particularly related to information management and communication, infrastructure development, and economics.

The advocacy function of the INS or IN also encompasses consumer health. INs may be part of initiatives such as promoting the adoption of technology for rural programs to increase access to health services. Advocacy may include educating legislators about increasing telecommunication access, expanding reimbursement for technology-enabled consumer services, or educating the public on ways to access health-related materials via the Internet. Examples of policy development and advocacy function of the INS or IN might include:

- The president of a health information management organization represents nursing on a national information standards task force.

- A lobbyist participates in advocacy efforts on behalf of consumers for increased government funding of demonstration or pilot informatics projects.

- A president of a nursing informatics organization writes letters to elected officials to obtain their support for reimbursement of services by remote, technology-enabled providers.

Research and Evaluation

INSs conduct research into the design, development, and implementation of informatics solutions, and their impact on users, such as healthcare organizations, providers, consumers, and payers. INS researchers use systematic methods of inquiry (including traditional and newer techniques) to identify and evaluate data, information, knowledge, and wisdom in informatics solutions and data repositories. Research and evaluation functions include, but are not limited to:

- Research in concept or symbolic representation of nursing phenomena
- Evaluation of clinical decision-making in nursing
- Applied research in development, implementation, usability, and outcome implications of solutions
- Consumers' and interdisciplinary providers' use of health information tools and resources
- Evaluation of effective methods for information systems implementation, acceptance, and utilization
- Human factors or ergonomics research into the design of systems and their impact on interdisciplinary providers, consumers, nurses, and their interactions
- Evaluation research on the effects of systems on the processes and outcomes of consumer care
- Usability testing of nursing and consumer applications
- Evaluating how consumers utilize computerized healthcare products
- Research in clinical vocabularies
- Interaction of consumers, providers, and technology
- Consumer communication and usage of technology-based support groups

Research in nursing informatics can span a range of activities, from experimental research to process improvement and informal evaluation to evidence-based practice. Much of the work is innovative and may be initiated by INSs or conducted at the request of an organization or agency. INSs working in research and evaluation might conduct research projects to develop and refine standardized nursing vocabularies, or link nursing interventions to outcomes in large data sets. This work is essential in defining, describing, and evaluating data, information, knowledge, and wisdom. It may include the evaluation of organizational attributes for successful adoption of documentation systems or the impact and efficacy of hardware and software solutions.

Nursing informatics research may also incorporate a consumer orientation. It may study effective nurse-consumer interactions in web-based interactions with older consumers, or the impact of new applications on nurses' workflow. Patient reactions to instant messaging from providers may be studied. Examples of the research function of the INS include:

- The chief for nursing research for a large software company oversees projects to evaluate the impact of enterprise electronic health records on patient care outcomes.

- A nursing informatics analyst in a hospital IT department aggregates data about the incidence of decubiti, creates trend reports and predictive models for nurse managers, and analyzes outcomes against quality indicators.

- A nurse researcher conducts a usability study comparing consumer entry of information at a clinic-based kiosk to in-person interviews.

Integrated Functional Areas: Telehealth and Telenursing as Exemplar

Informatics solutions are foundational support for healthcare delivery. In some cases, however, informatics solutions are more tightly integrated with care delivery. Clinical care and informatics intersect in areas such as telehealth and radiation oncology and serve as examples of integrated functional areas. In the discussion below, telehealth serves as the exemplar.

Telehealth, as defined by the U.S. Office for the Advancement of Telehealth, is "the use of electronic information and telecommunications technologies to support long-distance clinical healthcare, patient and professional health-related education, public health and health administration" (HRSA, 2001). Telenursing is the use of distance or telecommunications technologies by nurses to monitor consumer and public health and administrative functions, as well as deliver healthcare education (Milholland, 2000; NCSNB, 2003). With the widespread expansion of telehealth technologies, standards have been developed that take into account differing countries' cultures and governance standards

(Milholland-Hunter, 2001). Standards may pertain to the transmission of data and information as well as protocols for providing care.

Nursing informatics primarily fulfills a clinical support role, as opposed to a direct clinical practice role. Telehealth is primarily a clinical practice role, with technical aspects required to deliver care. The 2004 International Telenursing Survey (Grady, Schlachta-Fairchild, & Elfrink, 2005) surveyed international telenurses worldwide. Of the 719 participants, only 18 had informatics in their job titles. Within this group, over half were advanced practice clinicians. Ten of the clinicians had the term informatics in their titles. Thus, the interface between nursing informatics and telehealth nursing today primarily occurs at the technical or support level. In the future, telehealth may evolve toward an emphasis on information (versus technology), and informatics principles, methods, and tools may expand in the future.

Standards for telehealth nursing clinical practice are outlined in *ANA's Core Principles on Telehealth* (1998) and *Competencies for Telehealth Technologies in Nursing* (1999). These describe the interface between telehealth and informatics, referring to the technical aspects of telehealth as clinical support and telehealth as clinical practice. Examples of the telehealth role of the IN or INS might be:

- A telehealth network coordinator for a rural telehealth program ensures the appropriate deployment of technology, and customization for distance-related needs.

- A program manager for telehealth in a home health agency organizes the integration of telehealth into the agency's operations, supports the alignment of telehealth technology with the overall technology strategy of the agency, leads the adoption and implementation of the program, and evaluates and maintains telehealth outcomes and accountability for those outcomes (Starren et al., 2005).

- A nurse researcher conducting a program evaluation compares the impact of an online, telehealth cardiac education program to that of an in-person support group on level of depression and adherence to diet.

NI Functional Areas: Conclusions

With the continued miniaturization of technology, as well as developments in information science and nursing science, NI functions will continue to expand, evolving into functions not yet envisioned. INSs and INs will need to continually assess new knowledge management and technology trends and incorporate them into their own practices. Integrated functional areas will continue to expand. The functional areas listed here will be combined with new areas to create innovative positions of the future.

References: Functional Areas

American Medical Informatics Association (AMIA). (2006a). Nursing Informatics Working Group. *Roles in nursing informatics.* Retrieved October 10, 2007 from http://www.amia.org/mbrcenter/wg/ni/roles/inf_nrs.asp

American Nurses Association (ANA). (1998). *Core principles on telehealth.* Washington, DC: American Nurses Publishing.

American Nurses Association (ANA). (1999). *Competencies for telehealth technologies in nursing.* Washington, DC: American Nurses Publishing.

American Nurses Association (ANA). (2000). *Scope and standards of practice for nursing professional development.* Washington, DC: American Nurses Publishing.

American Nurses Association (ANA). (2004a). *Nursing scope and standards of practice.* Silver Spring, MD: Nursesbooks.org.

American Nurses Association (ANA). (2004b). *Scope and standards for nurse administrators* (2nd ed.). Silver Spring, MD: Nursesbooks.org.

Bellinger, G., Castro, D., & Mills, A. (2004). Data, information, knowledge, and wisdom. Retrieved October 10, 2007 from http://www.systems-thinking.org/dikw/dikw.htm

Center for Nursing Classification and Clinical Effectiveness (CNCCE). (2004). *Overview of NIC/NOC.* Retrieved October 10, 2007 from http://www.nursing.uiowa.edu/excellence/nursing_knowledge/clinical_effectiveness/index.htm

General Services Administration (GSA). (2006). Office of Government-wide Policy, IT Accessibility & Workforce Division (ITAW). *Section 508*. Retrieved October 10, 2007 from http://www.section508.gov.

Fayyad, U. (1996). Data mining and knowledge discovery: Making sense out of data. *IEEE Expert 11*(5), 220–225. Retrieved December 13, 2007, from http://www.aaai.org/AITopics/assets/PDF/AIMag17-03-2-article.pdf.

Grady, J., Schlachta-Fairchild, L. & Elfrink, V. (2005). Results of the 2004 International Telenursing Survey. *Telemedicine and e-Health, 11*(2), 197.

Greene, J. (2004). RN to CIO: High-tech nurses bridge hospitals' cultural divide. *Hospitals and Health Networks 78*(2):40–46.

Hammond, W.E. (1995). *Glossary for healthcare standards*. Retrieved February 28, 2006 from http://dmi-www.mc.duke.edu/dukemi/acronyms.htm.

Health Insurance Portability and Accountability Act of 1996 (HIPAA). Retrieved October 10, 2007 from http://aspe.hhs.gov/admnsimp/pl104191.htm.

Health Resources and Services Administration (HRSA). (2001). Office for the Advancement of Telehealth. *Report to Congress on telemedicine*. Retrieved October 10, 2007 from http://www.hrsa.gov/telehealth/pubs/report2001.htm.

Healthcare Information and Management Systems Society (HIMSS). (2007). *2007 HIMSS nursing informatics survey*. Retrieved October 10, 2007 from http://www.himss.org/content/files/surveyresults/2007NursingInformatics.pdf.

Milholland, K. (2000). *Telenursing, telehealth. Nursing and technology advance together*. Geneva: International Council of Nurses.

Milholland-Hunter, K. (2001). *International professional standards for telenursing programmes*. Geneva: International Council of Nurses.

National Council of State Boards of Nursing (NCSBN). (2003). *Position paper on telenursing: A challenge to regulation.* Retrieved October 10, 2007 from http://www.ncsbn.org/pdfs/TelenursingPaper.pdf

National Library of Medicine (NLM). (2006). *Unified Medical Language System.* Retrieved October 10, 2007 from http://www.nlm.nih.gov/research/umls.

Newbold, S. K. (2006). Nursing informatics database—Job titles as of January 17, 2006. Electronic correspondence. Email to snewbold@umaryland.edu.

Sensmeier, J., West, L., & Horowicz, J.K. (2004). Survey reveals, role, compensation of nurse informaticists. *Computers, Informatics, Nursing 22*(3), 171, 178–181.

Staggers, N, & Lasome, C. F. (2005). RN, CIO: An executive informatics career. *Computer, Informatics, Nursing 23*(4), 201–206.

Starren, J., Tsai, C., Bakken, S., Aidala, A., Morin, P., Hilliman, C., et al. (2005). The role of nurses installing telehealth technology in the home. *Computers, Informatics, Nursing, 23*(4), 181–189.

Willson, D., Bjornstad, G., Lussier, J., Matney, S., Miller, S., Nelson, N., et al. (2000). Nursing informatics career opportunities. In B. Carty (ed.), *Nursing informatics: education for practice.* New York: Springer.

Informatics Competencies

Because of the increased visibility of information and technology in healthcare settings and complementary educational programs, many stakeholders are faced with a need to define informatics competencies for nurses. Human resource managers and educational planners are just two examples of stakeholders who have an interest in competencies for nursing informatics.

Since 2000, researchers and professional organizations have completed substantial work in defining nursing informatics competencies (Androwich et al., 2003; Curran, 2003; Desjardins et al., 2003; HIMSS, 2005;

Jiang, Chen, & Chen, 2004; Staggers, Gassert, & Curran, 2000, 2001, 2002). Several lists of informatics competencies are available, especially those geared toward nurses' educational levels.

Stakeholders such as employers and educators are keenly interested in identifying informatics competencies for various nursing roles. For the discussion here, competencies for typical nursing informatics roles are especially pertinent. To this end, a matrix has been developed, based upon a thorough literature review and the work from a consensus panel. This text and accompanying matrix (Table 2) suggests competencies for typical nursing informatics functional areas discussed in the previous section.

The Intersection of Informatics Competencies and NI Functional Areas

Staggers, Gassert, and Curran (2000, 2001, 2002) studied the relationships between nursing roles and informatics competencies for nurses at four levels of practice: beginning, experienced, INS, and informatics innovator. This framework aligns with educational requirements for all nursing specialties at the beginning and experienced levels, and then identifies specific competencies for the specialty roles of INS and the informatics innovator. Their work not only promoted the integration of informatics competencies into educational curricula, but also influenced policy documents.

To date, the majority of authors have focused on the competencies needed for nursing curricula. Curran (2003) identified informatics competencies for nurse practitioners at Columbia University School of Nursing. Desjardins, Cook, Jenkins, and Bakken (2005) focused on beginning nurse competencies, expanding them to include the knowledge and skills for information literacy to support evidenced-based practice. Like Staggers et al. (2002), this study also linked competencies to four levels of nursing practice. Barton (2005) presented a similar view of informatics competencies for the beginning nurse, identifying a need for competencies in technology or computer literacy as well as information literacy for undergraduate nursing programs.

McNeil, Elfrink, Pierce, Beyea, Bickford, and Averill (2005) examined educational content for required informatics competencies. They asked the deans and directors of 672 baccalaureate and above education programs to describe informatics content taught in their undergraduate and graduate programs. Twenty-five unique content areas were identified for undergraduate (i.e., beginning nurse) and graduate (i.e., experienced nurse) levels of practice. Among the top-ranked competencies for both programs were: a) accessing electronic resources, b) ethical use of information systems, c) evidence-based practice skills, and d) skills for computer-based patient records. The undergraduate program respondents more often identified basic hardware and software skills, whereas the graduate program respondents included competencies related to innovation and change theory, national health database knowledge, and general systems theory.

Jiang, Chen, and Chen (2004) surveyed Taiwanese nursing education programs ranging from non-vocational and vocational nursing programs to collegiate programs for two-, four-, five-year, and graduate-level programs. The authors identified seven domains of competencies and linked them to differing levels of nursing education in Taiwan. In contrast to work in the United States, they identified domains mostly related to computer versus information literacy, including hardware, software, and network concepts; principles of computer application; skills in computer usage; program design; limitations of the computer; personal and social issues; and attitudes toward the computer.

New categories and concomitant competencies for education, as well as practice, are also available. Androwich et al. (2003) described NI competencies needed to improve patient safety and expand nursing practice. Garde, Harrison, and Hovenga (2005) reported specific competencies for:

- Nursing informatics knowledge and skills (e.g., health information systems, electronic patient records, telehealth).

- Information technology knowledge and skills (e.g., programming principles, software development, methodologies and processes, system analysis and design, database design and management).

- Knowledge and skills in organizational and human behavior (e.g., project management, inter-professional communication, risk management, policies and procedures).

- Clinical and health-related knowledge and skills (e.g., evidence based practice, clinical guidelines, care pathways).

The Healthcare Leadership Alliance (HLA) announced the creation of the HLA Competency Directory in the fall of 2005. This directory (HLA,

2005) identifies 300 competencies across multiple healthcare management roles, categorized into five domains:

- Leadership
- Communications and relationship management
- Professionalism
- Business knowledge and skills
- Knowledge of the healthcare environment

This directory may be especially pertinent for interdisciplinary settings.

A New Competencies Matrix

The competencies matrix in Table 2 (on page 38 and 39) is derived from Staggers, Gassert, and Curran (2002) and other authors mentioned earlier, and from the ANCC NI Certification exam (ANCC, 2007). These competencies are categorized in three overall areas: Computer Literacy, Information Literacy, and Professional Development/Leadership. Computer literacy competencies relate to the psychomotor use of computers and other technological equipment (Barton, 2005). Information literacy competencies deal with information retrieval knowledge and skills: knowing when there is a need for information; identifying the information needed to address a given problem or issue; finding the needed information and evaluating it; organizing the information; and using the information effectively to address the problem or issue. (ALA, 2006). Professional development and leadership competencies refer to the ethical, procedural, safety, and management issues for informatics solutions in nursing practice, education, research, and administration.

The horizontal axis of the matrix is based on the four educational levels as well as the NI functional areas defined earlier. It is important to recognize that informatics competencies need to be integrated into all educational levels. The panel identified competency foci for each functional area indicated by an **X**. Competencies cross the different nursing informatics functional areas. Although each sub-heading includes more granular competencies beneath it, nurses would not necessarily be expected to achieve every competency within a sub-heading. The areas identified by the **X** merely indicate an area of emphasis.

The absence of an **X** does not mean that the skill is completely irrelevant to that role; rather it means that the skill may not be emphasized in a particular functional area or NI role. Nor is someone in a given role required to have every skill indicated. For example, a quality improvement (QI) specialist is an NI role that would stress the *Analysis* functional area. An Informatics Nurse Specialist working in a quality improvement area would require competency in many of the indicated computer literacy skills including administration, communication, desktop, systems, and quality improvement, but would not likely need the simulation skills identified in the matrix. However, a quality assurance specialist, listed in the same functional area, would need knowledge and skills about simulations, especially if the NI in this role worked in an institution using simulation for staff development or for a vendor using this product.

The Functional Area-Competency Framework provides an example of the nursing informatics competencies for different functional areas within NI roles. Telehealth, which may be seen as more of an integrative area rather than a stand-alone functional role, is included to reflect intersections with various competencies. The list is not exhaustive, but presents beginning guidance to the essential NI competencies across computer literacy, information literacy, and professional development skills and knowledge. Currently the competencies are at different levels. In the future they may be re-evaluated, expanded, or collapsed.

Competencies and Metastructures

The components of metastructures—data, information, knowledge, and wisdom—can be compared to the elements in the competencies matrix. Using a patient care example, the beginning nurse uses skills that rely on the ability to obtain data. Computer skills, data entry, and the use of the patient's electronic medical record are the major focus of their practice. The experienced nurse builds on this and applies basic computer skills to information.

The INS has expertise in nursing, as well as higher levels of computer literacy, information literacy, and professional development and leadership. This increased level represents knowledge in nursing informatics. The INS analyzes systems and processes in order to apply knowledge to patient care, administration, research, or education. Last, the informatics innovator has achieved a level of knowledge coupled with experience, a combination that exemplifies wisdom. Wisdom in informatics may be the creation of unique methods for system design or evaluation, or the political finesse to justify purchase of a system.

Table 2. Informatics Competencies by NI Functional Areas

Competency Categories	Knowledge and Skills	Beginning Nurse	Experienced Nurse	Informatics Specialist	Informatics Innovator	Administration	Analysis	Compliance & Integrity Management	Consultation	Coordination, Facilitation, & Integration	Development	Education & Professional Development	Policy Development & Advocacy	Research & Evaluation	Integrated Areas
Computer Literacy															
	Computer Skills—Administration	×				×	×	×	×	×		×			×
	Computer Skills—Communication	×	×			×	×	×	×						×
	Computer Skills—Data Access	×													×
	Computer Skills—Documentation	×	×									×			×
	Computer Skills—Education	×	×									×			×
	Computer Skills—Monitoring	×	×	×							×	×	×	×	×
	Computer Skills—Basic Desktop Software	×	×	×		×	×		×	×	×	×			×
	Computer Skills—Systems		×	×		×	×	×	×			×	×	×	
	Computer Skills—Quality Improvement		×			×	×		×	×		×			×
	Computer Skills—Research		×				×		×	×	×	×		×	
	Computer Skills—Project Management			×	×				×	×	×			×	
	Computer Skills—Simulation					×	×	×	×	×	×	×	×	×	×
Information Literacy															
	Informatics Skills—Evaluation		×	×	×	×	×		×	×	×	×	×	×	×
	Informatics Skills—Role		×	×		×	×		×	×	×	×	×		
	Informatics Skills—System Maintenance		×	×		×	×		×	×	×	×	×		×
	Informatics Skills—Analysis			×	×	×	×		×	×	×	×	×	×	×
	Informatics Skills—Data/Data Structure			×		×	×	×	×	×	×	×	×	×	×
	Informatics Skills—Design & Development			×	×	×	×	×	×	×	×	×	×	×	×
	Informatics Skills—Fiscal Management			×	×	×	×		×	×	×	×	×	×	×
	Informatics Skills—Implementation			×		×	×		×	×	×	×	×		×
	Informatics Skills—Management			×	×	×	×	×	×			×		×	×
	Informatics Skills—Programming			×		×	×		×		×				
	Informatics Skills—Requirements			×		×	×	×	×	×	×	×	×	×	×

(continues)

Table 2. *Continued*

Competency Categories	Knowledge and Skills	Beginning Nurse	Experienced Nurse	Informatics Specialist	Informatics Innovator	Administration	Analysis	Compliance & Integrity Management	Consultation	Coordination, Facilitation, & Integration	Development	Education & Professional Development	Policy Development & Advocacy	Research & Evaluation	Integrated Areas
Information Literacy															
	Informatics Skills—System Selection			×		×	×	×	×	×	×		×	×	×
	Informatics Skills—Testing			×		×	×			×	×	×	×		×
	Informatics Skills—Training			×		×				×	×	×	×		×
	Informatics Knowledge—Impact	×	×	×	×	×	×	×	×	×	×	×	×	×	×
	Informatics Knowledge—Privacy/security	×	×	×		×	×	×	×	×	×	×	×	×	×
	Informatics Knowledge—Systems	×	×	×		×	×	×	×	×	×	×	×		×
	Informatics Knowledge—Research		×	×				×	×	×	×	×	×		×
	Informatics Knowledge—Regulations			×		×	×	×	×	×	×	×	×	×	×
	Informatics Knowledge—Usability/Human Factors			×	×	×	×		×	×	×	×	×	×	×
	Informatics Knowledge—Education			×	×	×	×		×	×	×	×		×	×
	Informatics Knowledge—Models & Theories			×	×	×	×	×	×	×	×	×	×		
	Informatics Knowledge—Nursing Classification, Taxonomies, & Nomenclature			×	×	×	×	×	×	×	×	×	×	×	×
	System Lifecycle				×								×	×	
	Organization Change Management		×	×	×	×	×	×	×	×		×	×	×	×
	Systems Theory			×	×		×			×	×	×	×		×	×
	Management Science				×			×	×	×		×	×		×
	Standards for Privacy & Security	×	×	×	×	×	×	×	×	×	×	×	×	×	×
	Human Computer Interface			×	×		×			×	×	×	×		×	×
	Computer Assisted Instuction											×			
	Statistical Analysis			×	×	×	×				×		×		×	×
	Adapting information technology as a primary means of patient safety	×	×	×		×	×	×	×	×	×	×	×	×	×

Work in Progress

Work in NI competencies is evolving. There is no single consolidated list of competencies across educational levels, or a reference list of competencies for employers. Perhaps it is premature to cease all innovation, but the proliferation of lists can be confusing to the uninitiated.

In addition to numerous researchers, academics, and employers, many professional organizations are actively working toward identifying competencies for nursing informatics, such as:

- The American Medical Informatics Association (AMIA)'s 10x10 program (AMIA, 2006b).

- The AMIA Educational Workgroup.

- The HIMSS nursing informatics working group.

- An NLN Task Group on Informatics Competencies and subsequent initiatives (NLN, 2005a, 2005b).

- Technology Informatics Guiding Education Reform (TIGER, 2006).

NI Competencies: Conclusion

The work on informatics competencies has expanded greatly in the last five years. After the initial work of Staggers, et al (2001, 2002), numerous authors and agencies have now developed informatics competencies. The new competencies matrix (Table 2) matches competencies with typical NI functional areas. In the future, the rapid pace of technological change and generation of information and knowledge will present challenges for maintaining current and accurate competencies for nursing informatics. Faculty must understand competencies for nursing informatics to make NI an integral part of curricula and to stimulate research. Besides the educational arena, employers show a growing interest in competencies. More important, within the next few years, the multiple lists of NI competencies will benefit from consensus and consolidation.

References: NI Competencies

Alliance for Nursing Informatics (ANI). (2005). *Member organization report*. Retrieved October 10, 2007 from http://www.allianceni.org/doc/ANI_MemberOrgReport2005-06.pdf.

Androwich, I.M., Bickford, C.J., Button, P.J., Hunter, K.M., Murphy, J., & Sensmeier, J. (2003). *Clinical information systems: A framework for reaching the vision.* Washington, DC: American Nurses Publishing.

American Library Association (ALA). (2006). *Information literacy competency standards for higher education.* Retrieved October 10, 2007 from http://www.ala.org/acrl/ilcomstan.html.

American Medical Informatics Association (AMIA). (2006b). *Oregon health & science university biomedical informatics distance learning course.* Retrieved October 10, 2007 from http://www.amia.org/10x10/partners/ohsu.

American Nurses Credentialing Center (ANCC). (2007). *Informatics Nurse Certification.* Retrieved October 10, 2007 from http://www.nursecredentialing.org/ancc/cert/eligibility/informatics.html.

Barton, A.J. (2005). Cultivating informatics competencies in a community of practice. *Nursing Administration Quarterly, 29*(4), 323–328.

Curran, C.R. (2003). Informatics competencies for nurse practitioners. *American Association of Critical Care Nurses Clinical Issues, 14*(3), 320–330.

Desjardins, K.S., Cook, S.S., Jenkins, M., & Bakken, S. (2005). Effect of an informatics for evidence-based practice curriculum on nursing informatics competencies. *International Journal of Medical Informatics, 74*(11–12), 1012–1020.

Garde, S., Harrison, D., & Hovenga, E. (2005). Skill needs for nurses in their role as health informatics professionals: A survey in the context of global health informatics education. *International Journal of Medical Informatics, 74*(11–12), 899–907.

Healthcare Information and Management Systems Society (HIMSS). (2005). *HLA competency directory: ensuring future leaders meet the challenges of managing the nation's healthcare organizations.* Retrieved October 10, 2007 from http://www.himss.org/asp/ContentRedirector.asp?ContentId=65250.

Healthcare Leadership Alliance (HLA). (2005). *Competency directory.* Retrieved October 10, 2007 from http://www.healthcare leadership alliance.org/directory.htm.

Institute of Medicine (IOM). (2003). *Health professions education: A bridge to quality.* Washington, DC: National Academies Press.

Jiang, W., Chen, W., & Chen, Y. (2004). Important computer competencies for the nursing profession. *Journal of Nursing Research, 12*(3), 213–225.

Marin, H.F. (2005). Nursing informatics: Current issues around the world. *International Journal of Medical Informatics, 74,* 857–860.

McNeil, B.J., Elfrink, V.L., Pierce, S.T., Beyea, S.C., Bickford, C.J., & Averill, C. (2005). Nursing informatics knowledge and competencies: A national survey of nursing education programs in the United States. *International Journal of Medical Informatics, 74*(11–12), 1021–1030.

McNeil, B.J., & Odom, S.K. (2000). Nursing informatics education in the United States: Proposed undergraduate curriculum. *Health Informatics Journal, 6,* 32–38.

National League for Nursing (NLN). (2005a). *Core competencies of nurse educators with task statements.* Retrieved October 10, 2007 from http://www.nln.org/profdev/corecompetencies.pdf.

National League for Nursing (NLN). (2005b). *Task group on informatics competencies.* Retrieved December 4, 2006 from http://www.nln.org/aboutnln/AdvisoryCouncils_TaskGroups/informatics.htm

Saranto, K., & Leino-Kilpi, H. (1997). Computer literacy in nursing; developing the information technology syllabus in nursing education. *Journal of Advanced Nursing, 25,* 377–385.

Staggers, N., & Gassert, C. (2000). Competencies for nursing informatics. In B. Carty (Ed.), *Nursing informatics: Education for practice* (pp. 17–34). New York: Springer-Verlag.

Staggers, N., Gassert, C., & Curran, C. (2001). Informatics competencies for nurses at four levels of practice. *Journal of Nursing Education, 4*(7), 303–316.

Staggers, N., Gassert, C., & Curran, C. (2002). A Delphi study to determine informatics competencies for nurses at four levels of practice. *Nursing Research, 51*(6), 383–390.

Technology Informatics Guiding Educational Reform (TIGER). (2006). *TIGER Summit.* Retrieved October 10, 2007 from http://www.tigersummit.com/

The Integration of Nursing Informatics

As the use of technology increasingly becomes integrated into nursing and every nursing role, the boundaries between the roles of nurses and informatics nurses are becoming even more blurred. It becomes important to identify the commonalities along the practice continuum for nurses in all levels and specialties, and also the functions that make the practice of nursing informatics unique among nursing specialties. Information is central to healthcare delivery. All nurses must be skilled in managing and communicating information and are primarily concerned with the content of that information, but nursing informatics is especially concerned with the creation, structure, and delivery of that information: from the use of technology at the bedside to provide direct care, to giving the healthcare consumer point-of-need access to healthcare information, through exploiting the data underlying this information to create new nursing knowledge. This range in the use of information and technology can be visualized on a continuum as seen in Figure 4.

Figure 4. A Continuum of Integrating Information and Technology into Nursing Practice.

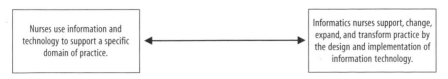

Nurses use information and technology to support a specific domain of practice. ⟷ Informatics nurses support, change, expand, and transform practice by the design and implementation of information technology.

Nursing informatics is also integrated into other healthcare informatics specialties. The INS is often responsible for implementing or coordinating projects involving multiple disciplines. The INS is expected to interact with professionals involved in all phases of the information systems lifecycle and with professionals in all aspects of system utilization. NI can be conceptualized either as an integral part of healthcare informatics or as a specialty within healthcare informatics. Core concepts are common to multiple informatics disciplines. There are also individual concepts and methods that are unique to one discipline. Two concept diagrams from Englebardt and Nelson (2002) demonstrate the different views of the role of NI in relation to other healthcare informatics specialties (see Figure 5).

NI is also integrated into all aspects of the healthcare continuum. This integration provides access to healthcare information at the point of need, such as at the bedside in acute healthcare settings, ambulatory care settings, at home, or even when traveling locally or globally.

Figure 5. The Healthcare Informatics Specialist: Two Models

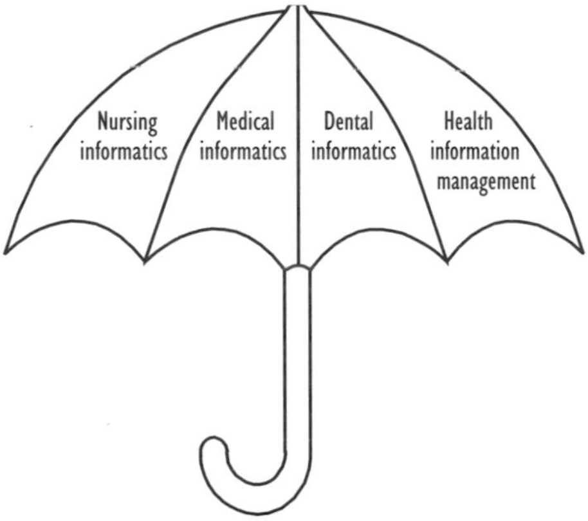

Umbrella Model 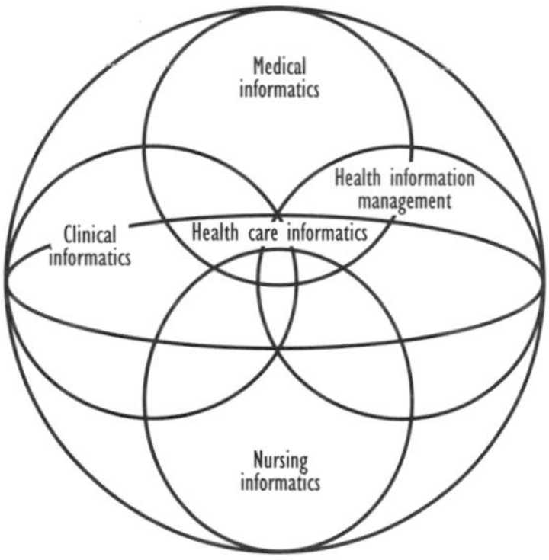   Overlapping Model

Reprinted with permission (Englehart & Nelson, 2002)

The Boundaries of Nursing Informatics

This section summarizes the differences between NI and other specialties in nursing, and between NI and other informatics specialties. To reiterate, NI is a specialty that integrates nursing science, computer science, and information science to manage and communicate data, information, knowledge, and wisdom in nursing practice. Critical thinking is a requirement of all nursing practice, and NI facilitates this critical thinking through the integration of data, information, knowledge, and wisdom to support patients, nurses, and other practitioners in their decision-making in all roles and settings. The difference between NI and other nursing specialties is the emphasis on informatics concepts, tools, and methods to facilitate nursing practice.

Although some outside the specialty might consider NI synonymous with information technology, technology alone does not define NI. The synthesis of data and information into knowledge and wisdom is central to NI, and information technology merely supports this process. INSs have adopted the anticipatory proactive stance characterized by Hannah, Ball, and Edwards (1994), and continuously strive to exploit technology in the design, structure, and presentation of information. They also consider the impact on healthcare delivery in general, and the nursing process specifically. Figure 6 illustrates the connection between the different foci of nursing and NI. These occur along a continuum without distinct boundaries.

Figure 6. Nursing and Nursing Informatics Foci

Nursing Focus	Nursing Informatics Focus
Nurses, patients, health, environment ⟶	Information user, information recipients, information exchange
Content of information, support for evidence-based practice changes ⟶	Design, structure, and representation of data as information
Using information applications and technology ⟶	Develop, implement, and evaluate applications and technology, ensuring the quality, effectiveness, efficiency, and usability of applications and technology

NI is also differentiated from other informatics specialties. Each informatics specialty is aligned uniquely with its primary role, requiring that INSs augment their base of nursing knowledge with unique informatics skills. Nursing informatics is recognized both as a component of the broad field of healthcare informatics and as a specialty within nursing (Brennan, 2002). This results in a unique body of knowledge and demonstrates the need for advanced preparation unique to nursing. NI incorporates informatics concepts used by others, but applies them to a foundation of nursing. What differentiates an INS or an IN from other informatics specialists is the knowledge of nursing content and process. The synthesis of informatics and nursing results in an integrated whole that is greater than its parts. Thus, an understanding of how informatics can support patient care in the context of the nursing process is fundamental to NI. Core components of informatics knowledge and skills underpin all informatics specialties, such as the use of technology, computer literacy, and data management structures. There are also components unique to each discipline such as their taxonomy.

Tenets of Nursing Informatics

- Nursing informatics contains a unique body of knowledge, preparation, and experience, and uses identifiable techniques and methods.

- Nursing informatics supports the clinical and non-clinical efforts of nurses and other providers to improve the quality of care and the welfare of healthcare consumers. Information or informatics methods alone do not improve patient care; rather, this information is used by clinicians and managers to improve care, information management, and patient outcomes.

- Nursing informatics collaborates with and is closely linked to other health-related informatics specialties.

- Although concerned with information technology, nursing informatics focuses on efficient and effective delivery of complete and accurate information in order to achieve quality outcomes.

- Human factors, human–computer interaction, ergonomics, and usability concepts are interwoven throughout the practice of NI.

- Nursing informatics promotes established, emerging, and innovative information technologies.

- The key ethical concerns of nursing informatics include advocating privacy and ensuring the confidentiality and security of healthcare data and information.

Ethics in Nursing Informatics

Nursing has a long history of applying ethical principles to nursing practice, with a primary concern for the patient and a commitment to the professional code of ethics for nurses. *Code of Ethics for Nurses with Interpretive Statements* (ANA, 2001) serves as a guide for the informatics nurse facing ethical issues, dilemmas, and decisions. The ANA policy on privacy and confidentiality (ANA, 2006b) addresses HIPAA legislation and the ethics of protecting information in a changing healthcare environment. Additionally, with the increase in electronic health records (EHRs) across multiple systems, decisions related to the use of information in the EHR must strike a balance between "ethically justified ends and otherwise appropriate means" (IMIA, 2006). The primacy of concern for patients and the commitment to this code of nursing ethics form a foundation for considering ethical issues in nursing, including nursing informatics. However, the practice of nursing informatics, a highly specialized and non-traditional nursing practice, also needs its own specialty-specific ethical guidelines.

Ethical questions often arise when common corporate business practices conflict with the ethical mandates of healthcare professionals. The INS brings an integrated, systems perspective to discussions of ethical issues, such as:

- Is a code of ethics integrated into the expanding distributed environment of electronic health information and healthcare service delivery?

- Is the individual responding to a healthcare related e-mail or web site inquiry appropriately licensed and qualified?

- In healthcare-related electronic communication, are appropriate safeguards in place to protect the sender's identity and privacy, the content and integrity of messages, and the respondent's identity?

The International Medical Informatics Association (IMIA) has published a detailed code of ethics for health information professionals. The IMIA code is meant to guide decision-making for "gathering, processing, storing, communicating, using, manipulating, and accessing health information" (IMIA, 2006). It offers ethical guidance uniquely applicable to nursing informatics. Among its general principles, two are of special interest to nursing informatics: information privacy and disposition, and legitimate infringement. The principle of information privacy and disposition states that all persons have a fundamental right to privacy, and hence control over the collection, storage, access, use, communication, manipulation, and disposition of data about themselves. However, the principle of legitimate infringement states that this fundamental right is tempered by the legitimate, appropriate, and relevant data needs of a free, responsible, and democratic society, and by the equal and competing rights of other persons.

Furthermore, INSs should understand and apply the basic principles of autonomy, beneficence, non-malfeasance, and justice as they relate to the practice of informatics (ANA, 2001). The INS encounters questions of biomedical ethics throughout systems development, implementation, and administration. For example, informatics professionals including nurse specialists must determine whether patients see all of their lab results online, perhaps before a clinician has seen them. This decision may be less a technical question than an ethical one concerning the principle of patient autonomy. Security standards respond to the principles of autonomy and non-malfeasance. In the United States, decisions concerning the appropriate access and use of data may be guided by both HIPAA rules and the ethical principle of justice.

The general principles described by the IMIA and ANA codes provide a solid ethical foundation for INSs. The INS has a responsibility to advocate for data confidentiality, integrity, and security, quality management of information, and legitimate data use. These needs must be balanced with users' timely access to accurate data for decision-making in all settings. The role of ethics in informatics practice is expanding, and INSs are in a unique position to make or share in decisions of informatics policy and operations. INSs can reconcile organizational risk with users' needs for timely data access. They can serve as the voice of wisdom—as translators and advocates for users who also understand the relevant ethical, political, and technological considerations.

New computing approaches such as knowledge discovery, clinical data repositories (CDR), and data warehouses have already created new opportunities for the INS to apply ethical principles. Vast electronic stores of digitized personal data already exist. Contemporary organizations are grappling with complex issues like regulation of data access such that only appropriate data is visible only to appropriate users. As technologies evolve and data stores increase, the ethics of data use and protection will become increasingly intricate, requiring continual evaluation and monitoring. Informatics professionals must consider the following ethical responsibilities (IMIA, 2006):

- To ensure personal competence, integrity, diligence, and responsibility for all actions performed.

- To ensure that an electronic record, or the data contained in it, are used only for the stated purposes for which the data was collected or for purposes that are otherwise ethically defensible.

- To ensure that appropriate structures are in place to evaluate the technical, legal, and ethical acceptability of the data collection, storage, retrieval, processing, accessing, communication, and utilization of data in the settings in which they carry out their work.

- To ensure that healthcare professionals are informed about the status of the information services upon which users rely and must immediately advise users of any problems or difficulties that might be associated with or could reasonably be expected to arise in connection with these informatics services (IMIA 2006, p 6). (For example, processes such as phone trees for notification of system difficulties need to be addressed in both the planning and implementation of those services.)

In conclusion, the INS has the opportunity and responsibility to face the ethical ramifications of design, implementation, and utilization of healthcare information systems and data obtained through reporting mechanisms. The INS is challenged to balance the improvement of health care with individual privacy, security, and safety. Balancing the autonomy of patients and their health information against the just use of health information to benefit others requires thoughtful consideration across multiple levels. Given the complexity and challenge of making ethical decisions related to healthcare information systems, the INS must contribute to and act in accordance with a general understanding of the applicable ethical principles.

The Future of Nursing Informatics

Our discipline is rapidly changing: it will change even while this document is being printed. Three trends will likely influence the direction of this change: positions and competencies for nurses and informatics, technological aspects of the field, and changes in healthcare delivery and regulatory requirements.

Trends in Positions and Competencies for Nurses and Informatics

The boundaries between INSs, other nurses, and associated health informatics disciplines are blurring. As information and technology are further integrated into the workplace, nurses in all settings will gain informatics knowledge and skills. The number and complexity of informatics competencies for nurses will continue to escalate. Some informatics competencies ascribed to informatics specialists will likely transfer to mainstream nurses, and the level of competencies required for INSs will continue to expand. Thus, the baseline set of NI competencies required of nurses at all levels will rise.

In the last few years, new areas of nursing have been incorporated into nursing informatics. For example, nurses who heavily use information and technology, such as telehealth nurses, may be considered one type of IN. As others in nursing design, implement, and evaluate informatics solutions, the scope of nursing informatics will expand still more. Nursing informatics is becoming a world community with fewer distinctions and more commonalities among INSs everywhere.

The role boundaries between other health informatics roles and NI are less conspicuous than in the past. One of the centerpieces of NI practice is its cross-disciplinary nature, with INSs often leading cross-disciplinary projects to craft usable informatics solutions for use by many disciplines. INSs have assumed executive positions in the health informatics arena. INSs and their health informatics colleagues serve in many of the same positions, blurring boundaries while using a shared set of functions, skills, and knowledge. This trend will likely continue as professional informatics organizations define a shared set of core knowledge and skills required by all informatics specialties. Probably the clearest trend is evolving change in the functional areas for INSs, a continual move from a generic set of skills for any one discipline toward a shared set of competencies based on functional areas required to enact a particular position (i.e., clinical analyst, informatics executive, futurist, KDD researcher, or database developer).

Trends in Technology

Information technology is becoming commonplace in our daily lives as well as in health care. For the first time in history, a generation exists never having known a world without the Internet, cell phones, online social networks, blogs, and other electronic media. People raised on this technology will be entering the healthcare field as knowledge workers as well as consumers of healthcare delivery. Implications for NI are:

- New models of work and education for technologically sophisticated users who are less resistant to technology and in fact demand it.

- Adapting to users with less skill in face-to-face communications.

- Consumers with even greater expectations of accelerated information and technology implementation.

Several advances in technology will likely impact nursing informatics in the future. A number of these are outlined in the following sections.

Nanotechnology

Nanotechnology—microscopic technology on the order of one-billionth of a meter—will likely impact the diagnosis and treatment of many diseases and conditions (Gordon, Lutz, Boninger & Cooper, 2007). Some of the pending technologies that will affect INSs, clinicians, and patients may include:

- New methods for medication administration
  - Sensing patient's internal drug levels with miniature medical diagnostic tools circulating in patients' bloodstreams.
  - Chemotherapy delivered directly to a tumor site, reducing systemic side-effects.
- New monitoring devices for the home:
  - A talking pill bottle that lets patients push a button to hear prescription information.
  - Bathroom counters that announce whether it is safe to mix two medications.
  - A shower with built-in scales to calculate body mass index (Hong Kong Polytechnic University).

- Measuring devices in the bathroom to track urine frequency and output and upload these data to a system or care manager.

- Non-invasive blood glucose monitors to eliminate sticks; sensors to compute blood. sugar levels using a multi-wavelength reflective dispersion photometer (Hong Kong Polytechnic University).

Tools for managing public health concerns

The threat of terrorism and bioterrorism, and the need for improved disease management across traditional boundaries, drive the demand for new tools and solutions that will concern the INS. Partnership with public health professionals and the emergence of public health informatics is a response to the need for population management tools and early disease detection.

Devices and hardware

The increased miniaturization of devices will change where and how IT solutions will be deployed. No perfect hardware solution exists in the market today to address all diverse nursing workflows and mobile caregiver demands. An emphasis on ergonomics and human-computer interaction will lead to new solutions to support diverse workflow requirements.

New integrated technologies—cell phones, smart phones, PDA's, and multi-functional devices—will increase common access to health information. These solutions are becoming ubiquitous in daily life. They will change clinicians' and patients' expectations and their interactions with technology. In particular, providers will be challenged to know as much about new disease treatments and research findings as patients with these devices are.

Wearable computing

Wearable computing is a revolutionary paradigm that shatters myths about what computers are and how they should be used. A computer can be worn, much as eyeglasses or clothing are worn, and interactions with the user based on the context of the situation. With heads-up displays, embedded sensors in fabrics, unobtrusive input devices, personal wireless local area networks, and a host of other context sensing and communication tools, wearable computers can act as intelligent assistants or data collection and analysis devices.

Many of these devices are available now. Smart fabrics with embedded sensors have been on the commercial market since 2000 and are being used in shirts, gloves, and other clothing. These wearable computer and remote monitoring systems are intertwined with the user's activity so that the technology becomes transparent. Sensors and devices can gather data during the patient's daily routine, providing healthcare providers or researchers periodic or continuous data on the subject's health at work, school, exercise, and sleep, rather than the current snapshot captured during a typical hospital or clinic visit. A few applications for wearable computing include (OSNF, 2007):

- Sudden Infant Death Syndrome monitoring for infants
- Ambulatory cardiac and respiratory monitoring
- Monitoring of ventilation during exercise
- Monitoring rescue worker's vital signs
- Activity level of post-stroke patients
- Patterns of breathing in asthma
- Assessment of stress in individuals
- Arrhythmia detection and control of selected cardiac conditions
- Daily activity monitors
- Monitoring heat stress and dehydration

Wearable computing is applicable to workers as well as consumers or patients:

- Proximity badges and RFID (radio frequency identification) to track providers for workflow or allow log on to systems.
- Glasses with a heads-up display of vital signs or images without losing focus on the patient (MIT Media Lab, 2007).
- Bar code scanners that fit on a finger, or wrist-activated input devices.

Future developments for input methods may also apply to the healthcare market. For example, an "interface-free," touch-driven computer screen, manipulated intuitively with the fingertips, responds to varying levels of pressure. Another example is virtual keyboards using Bluetooth technology, in which a keyboard can be displayed and used on any surface (*ThinkGeek*, 2007).

Robotics

The use of robotics in patient care will expand. Robots have been used for many years to deliver supplies to patient care areas. Robotics enable remote surgeries and virtual reality surgical procedures. At Johns Hopkins, robots are being used as translators for patients (Greenback, 2007). Hand-assist devices help patients regain strength after a stroke (*Science Daily*, 2007). Robots are providing a remote presence to allow physicians to virtually examine patients by manipulating remote cameras (Cisco Systems, 2007). In the future, robots may also be used in direct patient care, for instance, to help lift morbidly obese patients.

Knowledge representation

As more and more electronic data become available for and about patients over their lifetime, clinicians will need advanced tools to help locate and synthesize this vast volume of data. New research will yield advances in displaying vast amounts of data to clinicians to optimize patient care and patient and clinician efficiencies while avoiding medical errors. NI may need more nurses trained in knowledge representation, semantic representation, and other knowledge areas. This also has implications for knowledge discovery in databases, data quality, and a continued emphasis on data standards and data quality

Nurses constantly make complex and diverse decisions in their daily practice. Decision-making must consider relevant evidence-based and patient-specific information. As nurse decision-making becomes more complex, the need for computerized clinical decision support will increase. In the absence of explicit evidence-based guidelines for nursing decisions, novel technologies will be necessary to synthesize evidence from the literature or induce models from clinical data. Knowledge discovery in databases could play an important role in the induction of clinical knowledge models.

Genomics

Advances in mapping the human genome and understanding individual DNA will have a dramatic impact on what we know about patients. These data, especially once they are integrated into EHRs or personal health records (PHRs), will lead to advances in customized patient care and customized medications targeted to individual responses to medications. Care and medication can be precisely customized to patients based on their unique DNA profile and how they have responded to medications and other interventions in the past. This will dramatically change how patients are managed for specific diseases and conditions, and extend into the prevention of some diseases.

The inherent complexity of customized patient care will demand computerized clinical decision support. Predictive disease models based on patients' DNA profiles will emerge as clinicians better understand DNA mapping. These advances have implications for a new model of care and for the INS's participation in the development of genomic IT solutions. More than ever, patients will need to be partners in this development. Genomics will lead to many specialized advances in care delivery and be linked to exact, individualized data within a personal health record (PHR). Subsequently, advanced disease management with the ultimate goal of disease prevention will be possible. This change has many implications for ethics as well as informatics. In fact, genomics competencies and curricular guidelines are available online (ANA, 2007)..

Educational technologies

Evolving teaching technologies are changing the education techniques used in the classroom, the lab, and the clinical setting. For example, patient care simulators allow students to run programmed care scenarios in a safe environment and provide innovative options for teaching critical thinking skills. Group learning tools such as clickers, used in interactive teaching, can change how students engage with class content as well as how they learn to function as members of a team (Michaelsen, Fink, & Knight, 2007). Distance education technologies such as web-based course management systems and the related student support services are challenging basic education concepts such as what academic resources must be included in a library collection or how a university defines a credit hour of education. Administrative information systems are automating basic university functions like admissions, registration, student record management, grant management, and financial aid, for example (Nelson et al., 2006). This automation is forcing institutions to review and in many cases to revise their educational policies and procedures. These technologies require a paradigm shift in knowledge delivery, which affects students, instructors, and course content.

In these modern educational settings, faculty, with little more than office applications for support, continue to manage large amounts of data about individual students, curricula, and accreditation. Comprehensive, enterprise-wide educational information systems that integrate administrative and academic functions are just beginning to provide educators with tools to manage all aspects of the educator role. As nursing informatics faculty become actively involved in the design, monitoring, and evaluation of these comprehensive systems, they will create the healthcare educational institutions of the future.

Traditional tuition models are a barrier to the globalization of education, but they are being slowly eroded. New educational models are already being created as universities reach students beyond their walls or create virtual educational experiences, e.g., partnering with other institutions to deliver classes to students across a region. Perhaps in the future, universities will partner with business entities and vendors to create other innovative models of education.

Curriculum design will change. Information is now generated and made available so quickly that baseline knowledge for students will evolve away from specific content to methods of finding accurate, current information and knowledge. Future students may not be evaluated on specific knowledge for one area or course, but instead be evaluated on their growth over time. The INS will be at the center of this union of informatics and new educational models because of its focus on managing information.

Tools for patient access to health information

Patients will continue to become stronger partners with providers, with increased accountability for their own care. This type of model will require solutions and patient education by clinical nurses and INSs to devise the best methods of care as well as solutions to monitor and maintain patients' health.

Expanded use of IT in nursing

Technology use will increase everywhere in our work and home settings, perhaps even constantly traveling with us as wearable devices. Two implications are outlined here.

One is a current concern about students relying on available, structured information, computerized alerts, and reminders in systems such as EHRs and DSSs. Some educators and administrators now are concerned that if students rely on available, structured information, computerized alerts, and reminders in systems such as EHRs and DSSs, their critical thinking skills may diminish. Future INSs and educators will determine and test new academic and practice models. Perhaps academic applications will be designed differently than practice applications designed to encourage questioning and active cognitive engagement. Or system designers may need to modify systems to promote a different cognitive engagement by practitioners. Or educators may teach a new level of human information processing to maximize human capabilities, one beyond students needing to memorize structures for a physical examination and similar static information stored in an EHR. In this model, information technology serves as an aid to, not a replacement for, human thinking and judgment.

Reliability is the other implication of the increasing pervasiveness of IT. As applications are increasingly integrated into healthcare, the impact of downtime becomes more severe and quick recovery methods imperative. Especially with order management in place, institutions must ensure continuous business operations with uninterrupted access to applications and data. Strategies and technologies to support continuous uptime are available, and the INS is typically involved in defining, designing, and installing them. Pervasive computing creates a new standard for information access even when there is no power supply, like a laptop powered by a hand crank (OLPC, 2007). Thus, INSs must be strong advocates for systems to be continuously available. Likewise, they can be intimately involved in disaster recovery, including being an advocate for funding allocations for recovery methods.

In 2005, Hurricane Katrina emphasized the importance of redundant systems and effective disaster recovery procedures. Requirements for current and future systems will focus on prevention rather include reaction as well as these features:

- 24×7 operation and performance with redundancies throughout the system, failovers, and tested high reliability.

- Tools to assist in monitoring and managing the IT environment, monitor system use, and identify technology issues before system failure occurs.

- Scalable IT solutions as more clinical applications come online.

- Solutions that IT departments can manage without in-depth technology expertise.

Implications for INSs

INSs will need to have a systematic method for becoming aware of emerging technologies and their projected impact(s) to healthcare and informatics. INSs can be essential leaders and partners for the safe and intelligent incorporation of new technology and techniques into health informatics solutions. The content or information on devices is still the most critical component, and INSs can serve as content designers. Areas such as genomics may have ethical ramifications, and INSs must ensure that they are respected. Sub-specialization within NI will continue, and INSs may find themselves specializing in the safe use of particular technologies.

All of these areas have implications for curricular design and education. The expansion of technology amplifies the need for continuous availability of systems. On the other hand, the "digital divide" in large remains: a significant number of people have little access to information technology. INSs can also take the lead in eliminating the digital divide between those with access to information and those without. In all situations, INSs can advocate and apply methods for users to learn and use new technologies effectively and safely.

Trends in Healthcare Delivery and Regulation

One force that has driven information technology and EHR installations in the United States is a national emphasis on patient safety, including technology installation as a focal point for reducing errors in healthcare. Also responsible is the fact that health organizations such as AHRQ and IHI, as well as non-health organizations like Leapfrog, are impatient with slow progress, to the point that they are providing incentives for health institutions to implement informatics solutions. Other forces will likely escalate the pace of adoption. Organizations are using value-versus-return-on-investment models to justify health IT and pay-for-performance models will likely accelerate EHR installations. Data are becoming more visible to consumers and hospital boards. Organizations will continue to increase the transparency of data and, more importantly, improve the care being delivered.

Regulatory requirements and standards will shape the future. INSs will be involved in defining these and future standards, and in designing, building, implementing, using, and certifying products that comply. A number of projects are underway, among them:

- Certification Commission for Healthcare Information Technology (CCHIT). "CCHIT is a recognized certification body (RCB) for electronic health records and their networks, and an independent, voluntary, private-sector initiative." Their mission is "to accelerate the adoption of health information technology by creating an efficient, credible, and sustainable product certification program." (CCHIT, 2007)

- HL7 is defining interoperability standards for systems.

- The IEEEP2407 working group is developing standards for personalized health informatics.

- The Joint Commission continues to expand regulatory compliance for patient safety, e.g., national patient safety goals, medication reconciliation, and other requirements with implications for the INS.

- The Health Information Technology Standards Panel (HITSP) is harmonizing industry-wide health IT standards.

- The Nationwide Health Information Network (NHIN) initiative is creating prototype architectures for widespread health information exchange.

- The FDA (Food and Drug Administration) has several initiatives underway:
  - Bar code label requirements for human drug products and biological products (FDA, 2007a).
  - Draft guidelines for the safe and effective use of radio frequency devices.
  - Nanotechnology development (FDA, 2007b) and potential expansion of products covered, e.g., advanced decision support tools and similar informatics applications.

Care delivery models

Care is no longer a local phenomenon. Patients in rural ICUs can be monitored remotely by intensivists and ICU nurses. Pharmacists can provide remote pharmacological assistance to rural areas. Radiologists can read images in real time from anywhere in the world. Physicians are assisted by robots as they examine patients in distant locations.

Care is no longer limited to traditional healthcare settings, even when it is delivered locally. Clinicians are now available in retail stores, work settings, and other non-traditional places. These new settings will require new design, deployment, and support models that will challenge the NI specialist. INS involvement in the development of the robust health information infrastructure includes but is not limited to:

- Continued innovation of systems and expansion into less traditional settings such as long-term care and rural communities

- Personal health records will become more numerous. INSs will increasingly advocate for and assist patients with developing such individually maintained records. These can include one's own electronic vaccination history, past medical history, medications, allergies, condition, status, and visit history in an easily accessible online format. Patients' online communication with healthcare providers will continue to increase, as well.

- Clinical data repositories and regional health information organizations will support accurate, timely, and secure transfer of patient data across care settings (ultimately across hospitals, clinics, pharmacies, laboratories, clinician office, long-term care facilities, and others).

Consumer informatics

Patients will become stronger partners with providers, with increased accountability for their own care and greater interest in access to their own EMR data. As consumers become more technically adept, they will consider their electronic healthcare data as necessary and accessible as their online banking information or stock transactions. Likewise, consumers will begin monitoring and managing the health of younger *and* older family members for whom they are responsible.

External partnerships

Healthcare will likely see non-traditional organizations entering the healthcare arena. For example, one company with an online application for individual, secure financial records is now investigating expansion into personal health records. Likewise, healthcare should create new, non-traditional partnerships. Perhaps a partnership with the video-gaming industry would also be fruitful for interactive EHRs and yield ideas for optimal user interfaces.

Implications for INSs

New care models have vast implications for informatics nurses. These new delivery models will require INSs to continue developing informatics solutions for care in multiple, remote locations. INSs should have a key role in informatics solutions that emphasize quality care (McCormick et al., 2007). We need new models to shorten the time from design to installation in the systems life cycle. An 18- to 24-month build and implementation cycle is not tenable in an era of rapidly changing technology, care delivery, and expanding information access.

With the increasing number of information technology installations and the need to respond to burgeoning regulatory requirements, INSs will be at centerstage for all phases of the systems lifecycle. They will be developing and implementing new informatics solutions, ensuring data quality for implemented solutions, and evaluating the impact of solutions. The new model of consumer informatics will require technical solutions and patient education jointly from clinical nurses and INSs. INSs will need to devise the best methods of care as well as designing solutions that enable patients to monitor and maintain their own health. INSs will play a key role in designing new tools for data capture and analyses to comply with regulatory guidelines.

NI Future and Trends: Conclusions

The positions and competencies of nurses, changes in technology, and new trends in health delivery and regulation will shape the future of nursing informatics. Important concepts underlying these trends:

- Preparing for and evolving with new information and technology changes.

- Inventing and delivering new educational models to teach both new and existing nursing professionals.

- Designing, developing, implementing, and evaluating solutions for new information technologies across all areas of nursing and health settings.

- Incorporating newer technologies and methods to redesign care, research and administrative processes.

- Pioneering, designing, and facilitating changes in care models as they evolve away from episodic care toward more predictive and preventive models.

- Focusing on usability—designing and evaluating how information is presented to promote ease of use and adoption (human–computer interaction).

The global nature of informatics is already clear. In the future, care models and data will be shared even more widely. New technologies will create wider access to information and the need for a new generation of data and information management skills, analytic tools, new educational models, and different cognitive skills. Traditional boundaries of institutions, care delivery, and education will continue to erode. New positions and functional areas are emerging. Increased collaboration among NI colleagues and a shared scope and standard of NI practice will be the hallmark of the future.

References: Future and Trends

Certification Commission for Healthcare Information Technology (CCHIT). (2007). Home page. Retrieved October 10, 2007 from http://www.cchit.org/

Cisco Systems. (2007). Telemedicine pioneer helps physicians on the move stay close to patients. Retrieved October 10, 2007 from http://www.cisco.com/application/pdf/en/us/guest/netsol/ns554/c647/cdccont_0900aecd804073a3.pdf

Food and Drug Administration (FDA). (2007a). *FDA rule requires bar codes on drugs and blood to help reduce errors.* Retrieved October 10, 2007 from http://www.fda.gov/oc/initiatives/barcode-sadr/

Food and Drug Administration (FDA). (2007b). *FDA nanotechnology task force report.* Retrieved October 10, 2007 from www.fda.gov/nanotechnology.

Gordon, A.T., Lutz, G.E., Boninger, M.L., & Cooper, R.A. (2007). Introduction to nanotechnology: potential applications in physical medicine and rehabilitation. *American Journal of Physical Medicine & Rehabilitation*, *86*(3), 225– 241.

Greenback, L. (2007). Robot aids Johns Hopkins patients. *The Baltimore Examiner*. Retrieved January 9, 2007 from http://www.examiner.com/a-498079~Robot_aids_Johns_Hopkins_patients.html.

McCormick, K.A., Delaney, C.J., Brennan, P.F., Effken, J.A., Kendrick, K., Murphy, J., et al. (2007). Guideposts to the future—An agenda for nursing informatics. *Journal of the American Medical Informatics Association*, *14*(1), 19–24.

Massachusetts Institute of Technology (MIT) Media Lab. (2007). *Wearable computing*. Retrieved October 10, 2007 from http://www.media.mit.edu/wearables.

Michaelsen, M., Fink, L, & Knight, A. (2007) Team based learning: The power of teams for powerful learning. Retrieved October 10, 2007 from http://www.ou.edu/idp/teamlearning/

Nelson, R., & Ball, M. (Eds.). (2004) *Consumer informatics: Applications and strategies in cyber healthcare.* New York: Springer Verlag.

Nelson, R., Meyer, L., Rizzolo, M.A., Rutar, P., Proto, M.B., & Newbold, S. (2006). The evolution of educational information systems and nurse faculty roles. *Nursing Education Perspectives*. *27*(5), 189–195.

Offray Specialty Narrow Fabrics (OSNF). (2007). *Smart textiles*. Retrieved October 10, 2007 from http://www.osnf.com/p_smart.html

One Laptop per Child (OLPC). (2007). *A $100 laptop for the world's children's education*. Retrieved October 10, 2007 from http://www.laptop.org/

Science Daily. (2007). *Robotic brace aids stroke recovery*. Retrieved October 10, 2007 from http://www.sciencedaily.com/releases/2007/03/070321105223.htm

ThinkGeek. (2007). *Bluetooth Laser Virtual Keyboard*. Retrieved October 10, 2007 from http://www.thinkgeek.com/computing/input/8193/

Mendelson, H. (2005). *Moore's law*. Retrieved October 10, 2007 from http://www.thocp.net/biographies/papers/moores_law.htm

STANDARDS OF NURSING INFORMATICS PRACTICE

Nursing informatics (NI) is the specialty that integrates nursing science, computer science, and information science to manage and communicate data, information, knowledge, and wisdom in nursing practice. Nursing informatics facilitates the integration of data, information, knowledge, and wisdom to support patients, nurses, and other providers in their decision-making in all roles and settings. This support is accomplished through the use of information structures, information processes, and information technology.

The goal of nursing informatics is to improve the health of populations, communities, families, and individuals by optimizing information management and communication. These activities include the design and use of informatics solutions and technology to support all areas of nursing, including, but not limited to, the direct provision of care, establishing effective administrative systems, managing and delivering educational experiences, enhancing lifelong learning, and supporting nursing research.

The standards of nursing informatics practice include two components: standards of practice and standards of professional performance. Each standard includes measurement criteria that provide more detail about the expected knowledge, skills, and abilities necessary to meet that standard. Some standards include additional measurement criteria specific to informatics nurse specialists and their role and practice.

The standards of practice are organized using a general problem-solving framework that closely models the language provided in *Nursing: Scope and Standards of Practice* (ANA, 2004) that describes the familiar nursing process of assessment, diagnosis, identification of outcomes, planning, implementation, and evaluation. The problem-solving framework supports all facets of informatics practice, helps to identify and clarify issues, and aids in the selection, development, implementation, and evaluation of informatics solutions. These steps are not mutually exclusive and may often overlap.

Informatics solution is a generic term used in this document to describe an application, product, method, tool, workflow change, or other recommendation an informatics nurse makes after identifying and analyzing an issue. An informatics solution may encompass technology and non-technology elements such as developing a database, purchasing a new computer application, creating a standardized nursing vocabulary, designing informatics curricula, creating a spreadsheet, tailoring an application to a particular environment, designing a research study to describe required informatics competencies, describing information flow in a process redesign, creating newly re-engineered processes, or creating a structure for information presentation.

The standards of professional performance also reflect the model language provided in *Nursing: Scope and Standards of Practice* (ANA, 2004). They have been re-ordered, and include one additional standard that addresses advocacy.

These standards of nursing informatics practice and their measurement criteria apply to *all* informatics nurses and their practices. The measurement criteria for the informatics nurse specialist reflect the higher expectations from this role and advanced level of practice.

Principles of Nursing Informatics Practice

Three overarching principles are inherent in every aspect of nursing informatics practice and should be considered by informatics nurses and informatics nurse specialists when reviewing the standards of practice.

The informatics nurse:

1. Incorporates theories, principles, and concepts from appropriate sciences into informatics practice. Examples of theories could include information, systems, and change theories. Principles and concepts could include project management, implementation methods, workflow analysis, process redesign, organizational culture, or database structures.

2. Integrates ergonomics and human–computer interaction (HCI) principles into informatics solution design, development, selection, implementation, and evaluation.

3. Systematically determines the social, legal, regulatory, and ethical impact of an informatics solution on nursing and health care.

STANDARDS OF NURSING INFORMATICS

STANDARDS OF PRACTICE

STANDARD 1. ASSESSMENT

The informatics nurse collects comprehensive data, information, and knowledge pertinent to the situation.

Measurement Criteria:

The informatics nurse:

- Collects data, information, and knowledge in a systematic and on-going process, such as with a needs assessment to refine the issue or problem, or with workflow analyses to examine current practice, workflow, and the potential impact of an informatics solution on that workflow.

- Involves the patient, family, nurse, other healthcare providers, and key stakeholders, as appropriate, in holistic data collection.

- Prioritizes data collection activities based on the immediate or anticipated needs of the situation.

- Uses appropriate evidence-based assessment techniques and instruments in collecting pertinent data to define the issue or problem.

- Uses analytical models and assessment tools that facilitate problem solving.

- Synthesizes available data, information, and knowledge relevant to the situation to identify patterns and variances.

- Documents relevant data in a retrievable format.

STANDARD 2. PROBLEM AND ISSUES IDENTIFICATION
The informatics nurse analyzes the assessment data to determine the problems or issues.

Measurement Criteria:

The informatics nurse:

- Derives the problems, needs, or issues based on assessment data.

- Validates the problems, needs, or issues with the patient, family, nurse, other healthcare providers, and key stakeholders when possible and appropriate.

- Documents problems, needs, or issues in a manner that facilitates the determination of the expected outcomes and plan.

STANDARD 3. OUTCOMES IDENTIFICATION
The informatics nurse identifies expected outcomes for a plan individualized to the situation.

Measurement Criteria:

The informatics nurse:

- Involves the patient, family, nurses, other healthcare providers, and key stakeholders in formulating expected outcomes when possible and appropriate.
- Considers associated risks, benefits, costs, current scientific evidence, environmental factors, and expertise when formulating expected outcomes.
- Defines expected outcomes in terms of the patient, patient values, ethical considerations, environment, organization, or situation with such consideration as associated risks, benefits, and costs, and current evidence-based knowledge.
- Includes a time estimate for attainment of expected outcomes.
- Develops expected outcomes that provide direction for all key stakeholders.
- Modifies expected outcomes based on changes in the status or evaluation of the situation.
- Documents expected outcomes as measurable goals.

Additional Measurement Criteria for the Informatics Nurse Specialist:

The informatics nurse specialist:

- Identifies expected outcomes that incorporate scientific evidence and are achievable through implementation of evidence-based practices.
- Identifies expected outcomes that maximize quality, efficiency, and effectiveness balanced with economy.
- Supports the use of clinical guidelines, such as but not limited to the integration of clinical guidelines into practice, information system and informatics solutions, and knowledge bases.

STANDARD 4. PLANNING
The informatics nurse develops a plan that prescribes strategies, alternatives, and recommendations to attain expected outcomes.

Measurement Criteria:

The informatics nurse:

- Develops a customized plan considering clinical and business characteristics and the environmental situation.

- Develops the plan in conjunction with the patient, family, nurse, other healthcare providers, key stakeholders, and others, as appropriate.

- Includes strategies in the plan that address each of the identified problems and issues, which may include strategies for the synthesis of data, information, and knowledge to enhance healthcare delivery.

- Provides for continuity within the plan.

- Incorporates an implementation pathway or timeline within the plan.

- Establishes the plan priorities with the key stakeholders and others as appropriate.

- Utilizes the plan to provide direction to healthcare team members and other stakeholders.

- Defines the plan to reflect current statutes, rules and regulations, and quality standards.

- Integrates current research and trends in the planning process.

- Considers the clinical, financial, and social impact of the plan.

- Uses standardized language, tools, and methodologies to document the plan.

- Participates in the design and development of interdisciplinary processes and informatics principles to address the situation or issue.

- Contributes to the development and continuous improvement of organizational systems that support the planning process.

- Supports the integration of clinical, human, financial, and technical resources to enhance and complete the decision-making processes.

STANDARD 5. IMPLEMENTATION
The informatics nurse implements the identified plan.

Measurement Criteria:

The informatics nurse:

- Implements the plan in a safe and timely manner.

- Documents implementation and any modifications, including changes or omissions, of the identified plan.

- Utilizes specific evidence-based actions and steps specific to the problem or issues to achieve the defined outcomes.

- Utilizes clinical, financial, technical, and community resources and systems to implement the plan.

- Collaborates with colleagues and other stakeholders to implement the plan.

- Implements the plan using principles and concepts of quality, project, or systems management.

- Fosters organizational systems that support implementation of the plan.

- Incorporates new knowledge and strategies to initiate change in informatics and nursing practices if desired outcomes are not achieved.

STANDARD 5A: COORDINATION OF ACTIVITIES
The informatics nurse coordinates activities.

Measurement Criteria:

The informatics nurse:

- Coordinates implementation of the plan, including activities and resources necessary to achieve desired outcomes.

- Synthesizes data and information to prescribe necessary system and environmental support measures.

- Documents coordination of the activities.

Measurement Criteria for the Informatics Nurse Specialist:

The informatics nurse specialist:

- Provides leadership in the coordination of interdisciplinary informatics activities.

- Coordinates system and community resources that enhance delivery of care across continuums.

STANDARD 5B: HEALTH TEACHING AND HEALTH PROMOTION AND EDUCATION

The informatics nurse employs strategies to promote health teaching, health promotion, and education for informatics solutions.

Measurement Criteria:

The informatics nurse:

- Identifies the need to integrate health content and learning resources into healthcare systems that address such topics as healthy lifestyles, risk-reducing behaviors, developmental needs, activities of daily living, and preventive self-care.

- Participates in the design, development, implementation, and evaluation of health promotion materials and health teaching methods appropriate to the situation and the patient's developmental level, learning needs, readiness, ability to learn, language preference, and culture. The informatics nurse focuses on the integration of these into informatics solutions.

- Contributes to the design, development, implementation, and evaluation of the educational content, materials, and teaching strategies in a holistic manner (psychosocial, cognitive, affective) needed for the continuing education and professional development programs necessary to implement the plan.

Additional Measurement Criteria for the Informatics Nurses Specialist:

The informatics nurse specialist:

- Synthesizes empirical evidence on risk behaviors, learning theories, behavioral change theories, motivational theories, epidemiology, and other related theories and frameworks when designing health information and patient education materials and programs.

- Designs health information and patient education appropriate to the patient's developmental level, learning needs, readiness to learn, and cultural values and beliefs.

Continued ▶

- Evaluates health information resources, such as the Internet, within the area of practice for accuracy, readability, and comprehensibility to help patients, family, healthcare providers, and others access quality health information.

- Creates opportunities for feedback and evaluation of the effectiveness of the educational content and teaching strategies used for continuing education and professional development programs.

STANDARD 5C: CONSULTATION

The informatics nurse provides consultation to influence the identified plan, enhance the abilities of others, and effect change.

Measurement Criteria:

The informatics nurse:

- Synthesizes data, information, theoretical frameworks, and evidence when providing consultation.

- Facilitates the effectiveness of a consultation by involving the stakeholders in the decision-making process.

- Communicates consultation recommendations that influence the identified plan, facilitate understanding by involved stakeholders, enhance the work of others, and effect change.

Additional Measurement Criteria for the Informatics Nurses Specialist:

The informatics nurse specialist:

- Develops recommendations and strategies to address and resolve complex issues and problems.

- Establishes formal and informal consultative relationships that can also provide professional development and mentorship opportunities.

STANDARD 6. EVALUATION

The informatics nurse evaluates progress towards attainment of outcomes.

Measurement Criteria:

The informatics nurse:

- Conducts a systematic, ongoing, and criterion-based evaluation of the outcomes in relation to the structures and processes prescribed by the plan and the indicated timeline.

- Includes key stakeholders and others involved in the plan or situation in the evaluative process.

- Supports the integration and use of evidence-based methods, tools, and guidelines linked to effective outcomes.

- Evaluates the effectiveness of the planned strategies in relation to the attainment of the expected outcomes.

- Uses ongoing assessment data to revise the problems and issues, the outcomes, the plan, and the implementation and evaluative processes as needed.

- Disseminates the results to key stakeholders and others involved in the plan or situation as appropriate.

- Documents the results of the evaluation.

Additional Measurement Criteria for the Informatics Nurse Specialist:

The informatics nurse specialist:

- Uses the results of the evaluation analyses to make or recommend process or structural changes including policy, procedure, or protocol documentation, as appropriate.

- Synthesizes the results of the evaluation analyses to determine the impact of the plan on the affected patients, families, groups, communities, and institutions, networks, and organizations.

STANDARDS OF PROFESSIONAL PERFORMANCE

STANDARD 7. EDUCATION
The informatics nurse attains knowledge and competency that reflect current nursing and informatics practice.

Measurement Criteria:

The informatics nurse:

- Participates in ongoing educational activities related to appropriate knowledge bases and professional issues.

- Demonstrates a commitment to lifelong learning through self-reflection and inquiry to identify learning needs.

- Seeks experiences that reflect current practice in order to maintain skills and competence in informatics practice and role performance.

- Acquires knowledge and skills appropriate to the specialty area, practice setting, role, or situation.

- Maintains professional records that provide evidence of competency and lifelong learning.

- Seeks experiences and formal and independent learning activities to maintain and develop clinical and professional skills and knowledge.

Additional Measurement Criteria for the Informatics Nurse Specialist:

The informatics nurse specialist:

- Uses current research findings and other evidence to expand knowledge, enhance role performance, and increase knowledge of professional issues.

STANDARD 8. PROFESSIONAL PRACTICE EVALUATION

The informatics nurse evaluates one's own nursing and informatics practice in relation to professional practice standards and guidelines, relevant statutes, rules, and regulations.

Measurement Criteria:

The informatics nurse's practice reflects the application of knowledge of current practice standards, guidelines, statutes, rules, and regulations.

The informatics nurse:

- Engages in self-evaluation of practice on a regular basis, identifying areas of strength as well as areas in which professional development would be beneficial.

- Obtains informal feedback regarding one's own practice from peers, professional colleagues, key stakeholders, and others.

- Participates in systematic peer review as appropriate.

- Takes action to achieve goals identified during the evaluation process.

- Provides rationales for practice beliefs, decisions, and actions as part of the informal and formal evaluation processes.

STANDARD 9. QUALITY OF PRACTICE
The informatics nurse systematically enhances the quality and effectiveness of nursing and informatics practice.

Measurement Criteria:

The informatics nurse:

- Demonstrates quality by documenting the application of the nursing process in a responsible, accountable, and ethical manner.

- Uses the results of quality improvement activities to initiate changes in nursing and informatics practice and in the healthcare delivery system.

- Uses creativity and innovation in nursing and informatics practice to improve care delivery.

- Incorporates new knowledge to initiate changes in nursing and informatics practice if desired outcomes are not achieved.

- Participates in quality improvement activities. Such activities may include:

  - Identifying aspects of practice important for quality monitoring.

  - Using indicators developed to monitor quality and effectiveness of nursing and informatics practice.

  - Collecting data to monitor quality and effectiveness of nursing and informatics practice.

  - Analyzing quality data to identify opportunities for improving nursing and informatics practice.

  - Formulating recommendations to improve nursing and informatics practice or outcomes.

  - Implementing activities to enhance the quality of nursing and informatics practice.

  - Engaging in the development, implementation, and evaluation of policies, procedures, and guidelines to improve the quality of practice.

Continued ▶

- Participating on interdisciplinary teams to evaluate clinical care or delivery of health services.

- Participating in efforts to minimize costs and unnecessary duplication.

- Analyzing factors related to safety, satisfaction, effectiveness, and cost–benefit options.

- Analyzing organizational systems for barriers.

- Implementing processes to remove or decrease barriers within organizational systems.

- Obtains and maintains professional certification if available in the area of expertise.

- Designs quality improvement initiatives.

- Implements initiatives to evaluate the need for change.

- Evaluates the practice environment in relation to existing evidence, identifying opportunities for the generation and use of research.

STANDARD 10. COLLEGIALITY

The informatics nurse interacts with and contributes to the professional development of peers and colleagues.

Measurement Criteria:

The informatics nurse:

- Shares knowledge and skills with peers and colleagues as evidenced by such activities as presentations at formal or informal meetings and professional conferences.

- Provides peers with feedback regarding their practice and role performance.

- Interacts with peers and colleagues to enhance one's own professional nursing practice and role performance.

- Maintains compassionate and caring relationships with peers and colleagues.

- Contributes to an environment that is conducive to the education of healthcare professionals.

- Contributes to a supportive and healthy work environment.

Additional Measurement Criteria for the Informatics Nurse Specialist:

The informatics nurse specialist:

- Participates on interdisciplinary professional teams that contribute to role development and, directly or indirectly, advance nursing, informatics practice, and health services.

- Mentors other registered nurses and colleagues as appropriate.

STANDARD 11. COLLABORATION

The informatics nurse collaborates with key stakeholders and others in the conduct of nursing and informatics practice.

Measurement Criteria:

The informatics nurse:

- Communicates with key stakeholders regarding the practice of nursing and informatics.

- Communicates with key stakeholders regarding the role of nurses and nursing within the domain of healthcare informatics and patient care delivery.

- Collaborates in creating a documented plan focused on outcomes and decisions related to the management of data, information, and knowledge for the delivery of healthcare services.

- Partners with others to effect change and generate positive outcomes through knowledge of the plan and situation.

- Documents plans, communications, rationales for plan changes, and collaborative discussions.

Additional Measurement Criteria for Informatics Nurse Specialist:

The informatics nurse specialist:

- Partners with others to enhance health care, and ultimately patient care, through interdisciplinary activities such as education, consultation, management, technological development, or research opportunities.

STANDARD 12. ETHICS
The informatics nurse integrates ethical provisions in all areas of practice.

Measurement Criteria:

The informatics nurse:

- Uses *Code of Ethics for Nurses with Interpretive Statements* (ANA, 2001) to guide practice.

- Uses nursing and informatics principles and methodologies in a manner that preserves and protects patient autonomy, dignity, and rights.

- Employs informatics principles, standards, and methodologies to establish and maintain patient confidentiality within legal and regulatory parameters.

- Evaluates factors related to privacy, security, and confidentiality in the use and handling of data, information, and knowledge.

- Promotes active engagement of community members in the oversight and management of the exchange of health information.

- Serves as a patient advocate assisting patients in developing skills for self advocacy.

- Contributes to resolving ethical issues of patients, colleagues, or systems as evidenced in such activities as participating on ethics committees.

- Reports illegal, incompetent, or impaired practices.

- Seeks available resources as needed when formulating ethical decisions.

- Demonstrates a commitment to practicing self-care, managing stress, and connecting with self and others.

Continued ▶

Additional Measurement Criteria for the Informatics Nurse Specialist:

The informatics nurse specialist

- Participates on multidisciplinary and interdisciplinary teams that address ethical risks, benefits, and outcomes.

- Informs administrators or others of the risks, benefits, and outcomes of programs and decisions that affect healthcare delivery.

STANDARD 13. RESEARCH
The informatics nurse integrates research findings into practice.

Measurement Criteria:

The informatics nurse:

- Utilizes the best available evidence, including research findings, to guide practice decisions.

- Actively participates in research activities at various levels appropriate to the nurse's level of education and position. Such activities may include:

  - Identifying clinical, nursing, and informatics problems or issues specific to nursing research.

  - Participating in data collection such as surveys, pilot projects, and formal studies.

  - Participating in a formal committee or program.

  - Sharing research activities and findings with peers and others.

  - Conducting research.

  - Critically analyzing and interpreting research for application to practice.

  - Using research findings in the development of policies, procedures, and standards of practice in patient care.

  - Incorporating research as a basis for learning.

Additional Measurement Criteria for the Informatics Nurse Specialist:

The informatics nurse specialist:

- Contributes to nursing knowledge by conducting or synthesizing research that discovers, examines, and evaluates knowledge, theories, criteria, and creative approaches to improve health care.

- Formally disseminates research findings through activities such as presentations, publications, consultation, and journal clubs.

STANDARD 14. RESOURCE UTILIZATION

The informatics nurse considers factors related to safety, effectiveness, cost, and impact on practice in the planning and delivery of services to achieve expected outcomes.

Measurement Criteria:

The informatics nurse:

- Evaluates factors such as safety, effectiveness, availability, cost and benefits, efficiencies, and impact on practice, when choosing practice options that would result in the same expected outcome.

- Assists stakeholders in identifying and securing appropriate and available services to address identified needs and implement and complete the plan or other activity.

- Assigns or delegates tasks based on the knowledge, skills, and abilities of the individual, complexity of the task, and predictability of the outcome.

- Assists stakeholders in becoming informed consumers about the options, costs, risks, and benefits of the plan and its associated activities.

Additional Measurement Criteria for the Informatics Nurse Specialist:

The informatics nurse specialist:

- Develops innovative solutions and applies strategies to obtain appropriate resources for nursing initiatives.

- Secures organizational resources to ensure a work environment conducive to completing the identified plan and outcomes.

- Develops evaluation methods to measure the safety and effectiveness of interventions and outcomes.

- Promotes activities that assist stakeholders, as appropriate, in becoming informed about costs, risks, and benefits of care or of the plan and solution.

STANDARD 15. ADVOCACY

The informatics nurse advocates for the protections and rights of patients, healthcare providers, institutions and organizations, and for issues related to data, information, knowledge, and health care.

Measurement Criteria:

The informatics nurse:

- Supports patients' access to their own personal health information within a reasonable time.

- Promotes patients' awareness of how their personal health data and information may be used and who has access to it.

- Supports the individual's right and ability to supplement, request correction of, and share their personal health data and information.

- Evaluates factors related to privacy, security, and confidentiality in the use and handling of health information.

- Promotes awareness and education of the healthcare consumer with regard to appropriate data collection, information sharing, information access, and associated issues.

- Supports patient involvement in their own care, facilitated by access to personal healthcare data.

- Promotes active engagement of community members in the development, oversight, and management of health information exchange.

- Educates clinicians, patients, and communities about the rights, responsibilities, and accountability entailed in the collection, use, and exchange of healthcare data and information.

- Incorporates the identified needs of the patient, family, healthcare provider, organization, and key stakeholders in policy development, program and services planning, and systems design.

- Integrates advocacy into the implementation of policies, programs and services, and systems for the patient.

Continued ▶

- Evaluates the effectiveness of advocating for the patient, family, healthcare provider, organization, and key stakeholders when assessing the actual outcomes.

- Demonstrates skill in advocating before providers and stakeholders on behalf of the patient, community, or population.

- Strives to resolve conflicting expectations from patients, families, communities, populations, healthcare providers, and other stakeholders.

Additional Measurement Criteria for the Informatics Nurse Specialist:

The informatics nurse specialist:

- Demonstrates skill in advocating on behalf of the patient, key stakeholders, programs, and services before public representatives and decision-makers.

- Exhibits fiscal responsibility and integrity in advocacy and formulating policy.

- Serves as an expert for patients, peers, other healthcare providers, and other stakeholders in promoting and implementing policies related to the management of data, information, and knowledge.

STANDARD 16. LEADERSHIP
The informatics nurse provides leadership in the professional practice setting and the profession.

Measurement Criteria:

The informatics nurse:

- Engages in teamwork as a team player and a team builder.

- Works to create and maintain healthy work environments in local, regional, national, or international communities.

- Displays the ability to define a clear vision, the associated goals, and a plan to implement and measure progress.

- Demonstrates a commitment to continuous, lifelong learning for self and others.

- Teaches others to succeed by mentoring and other strategies.

- Exhibits creativity and flexibility through times of change.

- Demonstrates energy, excitement, and a passion for quality work.

- Willingly accepts mistakes by self and others, thereby creating a culture in which risk-taking is not only safe, but expected.

- Inspires loyalty through valuing of people as the most precious asset in an organization.

- Directs the coordination of the plan across settings and among caregivers and other stakeholders.

- Serves in key roles in the work setting by participating on committees, councils, and administrative teams.

- Promotes advancement of the profession through participation in professional organizations.

- Assumes leadership roles within organizations representing nursing informatics professional practice in the healthcare domain.

Continued ▶

Additional Measurement Criteria for the Informatics Nurse Specialist:

The informatics nurse specialist:

- Serves in key leadership roles defining the vision, strategy, and tactical plans related to the management of data, information, and knowledge.

- Works to influence decision-making bodies to improve patient care, health services, and policies through such things as the adoption of data standards.

- Promotes communication of information and advancement of the profession through writing, publishing, and presentations for professional or lay audiences.

- Designs innovations to effect change in practice and outcomes.

- Provides direction to enhance the effectiveness of the interdisciplinary team and key stakeholders.

GLOSSARY

Beginning nurse. A nurse who is preparing for initial entry into nursing practice or has just begun a nursing career.

Computer literacy. The knowledge and skills needed to use basic computer applications and computer technology.

Data. Discrete entities that are described objectively without interpretation.

Decision support system (DSS). A computer application designed to facilitate human decision-making. Usually a DSS is rule-based, using a specified knowledge base and a set of rules to analyze data and information and provide recommendations.

Experienced nurse. A nurse with proficiency in one or more domains of practice.

Expert system. A type of decision support system that implements the knowledge of human experts.

Human-Computer Interaction. Study of the ways in which people, software applications, and computer technology influence each other.

Informatics Nurse Specialist (INS). A Registered Nurse with formal, graduate-level education in informatics or a related field; a specialist in the field of nursing informatics.

Informatics Nurse (IN). A Registered Nurse with an interest or experience in an informatics field; a generalist in the field of nursing informatics.

Informatics solution. The product an INS recommends after identifying and analyzing an issue. It may encompass technology and non-technology products such as information systems, new applications, nursing vocabulary, or informatics curricula.

Information. Data that are interpreted, organized, or structured.

Information Literacy. The ability to recognize when information is needed and to locate, evaluate, and effectively use that information.

Interdisciplinary. Reliant on the overlapping skills and knowledge of each team member and discipline, resulting in synergistic effects where outcomes are enhanced and more comprehensive than the simple effect of any individual team member's efforts.

Knowledge. Information that is synthesized so that relationships are identified and formalized.

Nursing informatics (NI). A specialty that integrates nursing science, computer science, and information science to manage and communicate data, information, knowledge, and wisdom in nursing practice. Nursing informatics facilitates the integration of data, information, and knowledge to support patients, nurses, and other providers in decision-making in all roles and settings. This support is accomplished through the use of information structures, information processes, and information technology.

Wisdom. The appropriate use of knowledge to solve human problems; understanding when and how to apply knowledge.

APPENDIX A.
Scope and Standards of Nursing Informatics Practice (2001)

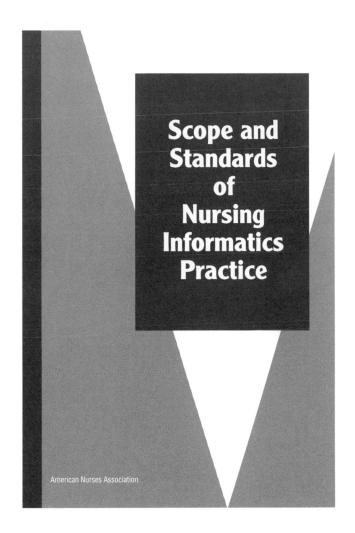

Scope and Standards of Nursing Informatics Practice

American Nurses Association

SCOPE and STANDARDS
of
Nursing Informatics
Practice

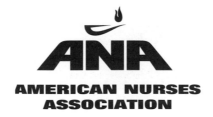

**AMERICAN NURSES
ASSOCIATION**

Library of Congress Cataloging-in-Publication Data

Scope and standards of nursing informatics practice.
    p. ; cm.
Includes bibliographical references.
   ISBN 1-55810-166-7
   1. Nursing informatics—Standards.
   [DNLM: 1. Medical Informatics—standards. 2. Nursing—standards. 3.
Medical Records Systems, Computerized. 4. Nursing—organization &
administration. 5. Nursing Records—standards. WY 26.6 S422 2001]
   I. American Nurses Association
   RT50.5 .S36 2001
   610.73′0285—dc21

                                     2001045885

Published by
Nursesbooks.org
8515 Georgia Avenue
Suite 400
Silver Spring, MD 20910

First printing Oct. 2001. Second printing May 2002. Third printing March
2004. Fourth printing August 2005. Fifth printing April 2006. Sixth printing
February 2007.

ISBN 978-1-55810-166-1
   (1-55810-166-7)

NIP21   .75M   02/07R

ACKNOWLEDGMENTS

American Nurses Association Workgroup to Review and Revise the *Scope of Practice for Nursing Informatics and the Standards of Nursing Informatics*

Nancy Staggers, PhD, RN, FAAN, Chairperson

Carole A. Gassert, PhD, RN, FAAN, FACMI

Jan Lee Kwai, MSN, RN,BC, CNOR

D. Kathy Milholland Hunter, PhD, RN

Ramona Nelson, PhD, RN,BC

Joyce Sensmeier, MS, RN,BC

Diane Struck, Lt Col (USAF), MS, RN,BC

John Welton, PhD, RN

ANA Staff

Carol Bickford, PhD, RN,BC

Winifred Carson, JD

Yvonne Humes, BA

The authors are very grateful to Judith Graves, PhD, RN, FAAN, for providing her insights and wisdom that enriched our discussions in the metastructure section of this document.

CONTENTS

INTRODUCTION

Nursing informatics is a specialty that integrates nursing science, computer science, and information science to manage and communicate data, information, and knowledge in nursing practice. Nursing informatics facilitates the integration of data, information, and knowledge to support patients, nurses, and other providers in their decision-making in all roles and settings. This support is accomplished through the use of information structures, information processes, and information technology.

The goal of nursing informatics is to improve the health of populations, communities, families, and individuals by optimizing information management and communication. This includes the use of technology in the direct provision of care, in establishing effective administrative systems, in managing and delivering educational experiences, in supporting life-long learning, and in supporting nursing research.

The purpose of this document is to delineate the scope of nursing informatics practice and the standards for the Informatics Nurse Specialist (INS). However, some sections of this work have application to the informatics needs of all nurses. This document expands on earlier work within nursing informatics (NI), providing historical as well as state-of-the-science material for the specialty (ANA, 1994, 1995). Because of the rapid changes in nursing, computer, and information sciences, NI role specifications, and thinking within informatics, a new document was needed. This revision provides new sections on metastructures and concepts underpinning NI, human–computer interaction, and ergonomics concepts; the evolution of NI definitions; a definition, goal, and role specification for NI; informatics competencies and the roles of the informatics nurse specialist; ethics in nursing informatics; and revised standards of practice.

This revised scope and standards document can be useful in several ways. First, the document outlines the attributes and definition of the specialty, differentiating it from other nursing specialties and validating NI as a distinct specialty within nursing. Second, the document can be useful to informatics educational programs and NI practitioners as a reference and guide. Third, this work can serve as a reference for employers; for example, to assist with developing of position descriptions. Last, the material can serve as a source document for funding agencies and others seeking to understand NI.

SCOPE OF PRACTICE OF NURSING INFORMATICS

Nursing Informatics

Nursing informatics (NI) is one example of a discipline-specific informatics practice within the broader category of health informatics. NI has become well established within nursing since its recognition as a specialty for registered nurses by the American Nurses Association (ANA) in 1992.

The specialty of NI is important to nursing and health care. It focuses on the representation of nursing data, information, and knowledge (Graves and Corcoran, 1989; Henry, 1995) and the management and communication of nursing information within the broader context of health informatics. Nursing informatics (1) provides a nursing perspective, (2) illuminates nursing values and beliefs, (3) denotes a practice base for nurses in NI, (4) produces unique knowledge, (5) distinguishes groups of practitioners, (6) focuses on the phenomena of interest for nursing, and (7) provides needed nursing language and word context (Brennan, 1994) to health informatics.

Specialty Attributes of Nursing Informatics

Panniers and Gassert (1996), who applied Styles' (1989) earlier work on specialization to informatics, discussed the following five attributes or characteristics that must be present to designate a specialty in nursing:

- A differentiated practice
- A defined research program
- Organizational representation
- Educational programs
- A credentialing mechanism

Differentiated Practice

The focus of nursing informatics (NI) separates or differentiates it from other specialties within nursing and from other discipline-specific specialties within health informatics. The nursing phenom ena of interest are the patient, health, environment, and nurse. Nurs ing informatics shares interest in these four phenomena, bu focuses on the structure and algorithms of data, information, anc knowledge used by nurses in their practice (Lange, 1997), whethe that practice is clinical, administrative, educational, and/or re search centered. Other specialties within nursing are concernec about the content of data and information, and less concernec about the structure of that data and information. Nursing infor matics is also charged with ensuring that nursing's data are repre sented and included in the computerized/electronic processing o health information.

For three decades or more, nurses have held informatics role and been key stakeholders in developing, implementing, and eval uating informatics solutions. Although implementing informatic solutions continues to be very important, more recently informatic nurse specialists have worked to develop and refine nursing's lan guage, implement telehealth systems, establish NI educational pro grams, and expand the focus of NI research, among other activities These examples reflect the diverse nature of NI practice. Because i is difficult to be an expert in each one of these informatics subspe cialties, informatics nurse specialists tend to focus their practice i one or two areas of NI. Subsequent discussions in this documen that define NI and its practice will expand this concept of differen tiated practice.

Defined Research Program

Research within nursing informatics (NI) is exceptionally varied However, the National Center for Nursing Research (NCNR) within the National Institute for Nursing Research (NINR), identi fied these specific research priorities for NI. Published by NIN] (then the National Center for Nursing Research), the seven priori ties for NI research were identified as follows (NCNR, 1993):

- Using data, information, and knowledge to deliver and manag patient care.

- Defining and describing data and information for patient care.

- Acquiring and delivering knowledge from and for patient care.

- Investigating new technologies to create tools for patient care.

- Applying patient care ergonomics to the patient–nurse–machine interaction.

- Integrating systems for better patient care.

- Evaluating the effects of nursing informatics solutions.

Most of the recommendations in the 1993 report are impacted by the development of nursing language. In other words, nursing language development and refinement have been seen as a cornerstone of NI research. Therefore, NI research funding has generally been focused in this area.

In 1998, survey results that describe more recent efforts to identify NI research priorities were presented at the international medical informatics meeting (Brennan et al., 1998). A sample of NI researchers across the country was surveyed in 1997 to identify NI research priorities, and to determine how similar or different these priorities were from those established in 1993 by NINR. Ten priorities were identified:

- Standardized language/vocabularies

- Technology development to support practice and patient care

- Data base issues

- Patient use of information technologies

- Using telecommunications technology for nursing practice

- Putting technology into practice

- Systems evaluation issues

- Information needs of nurses and other clinicians

- Nursing intervention innovations for professional practice

- Professional practice issues

In comparing the 1993 NINR report and 1997 survey responses, researchers found a substantial overlap between the two sets of priorities. The greatest emphasis continues to be on nursing language and the development of databases for clinical information. Both sets of priorities also list the need for developing and evaluating decision support tools and evaluating the impact of informatics solutions. Brennan et al. (1998) stated that the newer areas of interest were patients as users of information technology, telecommunications, and issues of privacy and confidentiality.

To date, obtaining funding for NI research in areas other than nursing vocabulary has been difficult. To secure funding, most NI researchers have linked projects to clinical priorities identified by funding agencies. For example, NI researchers could explore funding opportunities at NINR to examine the impact of telehealth systems on patient outcomes. Even though the availability of funding for NI research remains an issue, having a defined research agenda has helped to direct funding agencies and NI researchers. The research agenda has also allowed NI to meet the second required attribute of a specialty.

Organizational Representation

To qualify as a specialty, an area of practice must be represented by at least one organization. Nursing informatics (NI) is well-represented in several organizations at the international, national, regional, and local levels. For example, NI has a work group or special interest group in the American Medical Informatics Association (AMIA); International Medical Informatics Association (IMIA), an international organization; and many regional and local organizations. The NI groups have been essential in (1) establishing the scope of practice and standards of NI, (2) introducing the health informatics community to NI, (3) providing a forum for informatics nurse specialists to network and share issues and solutions, and (4) providing and participating in programs for professional development.

Educational Programs

The first two graduate programs in nursing informatics (NI) were established at the University of Maryland and University of Utah in 1988 and 1990, respectively. Both programs were funded by grants from the Division of Nursing, Health Resources and Services Administration (National Advisory Council on Nurse Education and Practice, 1997). From 1992 to 1998, changes in Title VIII legislation prevented federal funding of NI graduate programs. Because of funding restrictions, development of additional NI educational programs was slowed, but the emergence of NI programs has increased dramatically in the last few years. There is also an increasing interest in developing certificate programs that enable nurses who hold a master's degree to complete special course work in NI.

Some nurses have chosen to enter health informatics, medical informatics, or business programs to acquire needed informatics skills. The widening availability of degree-granting informatics programs has increased educational opportunities for nurses interested in informatics as a career (Gassert, 2000). Thus, the fourth characteristic of a specialty has been fulfilled.

Credentialing

A fifth attribute needed for acknowledging a professional specialty is the development of a certification mechanism. Scope of practice and standards documents for NI were developed under the direction of ANA in 1994 and 1995. These documents were then used by the American Nurses Credentialing Center (ANCC) as a foundation to develop an examination for nurses to become certified as generalists in NI.

Metastructures, Concepts, and Tools of Nursing Informatics

Metastructures are overarching concepts used in theories and sciences. Currently data, information, and knowledge are the metastructures in NI. Sciences underpinning nursing informatics (NI), concepts and tools from information science and computer science, human–computer interaction and ergonomics concepts, and the phenomena of nursing are also of interest in NI.

Metastructures: Data, Information, and Knowledge

In 1989, Graves and Corcoran published a classic work that describes the study of nursing informatics (NI). The article contributes two major thoughts to NI that will be acknowledged here. The first contribution is an information model that identifies data, information, and knowledge as key components of NI practice. Graves and Corcoran (1989) draw from Blum (1986) to define the three concepts as follows:

- *Data* are discrete entities that are described objectively without interpretation,

- *Information* is data that are interpreted, organized, or structured, and

- *Knowledge* is information that is synthesized so that relationships are identified and formalized.

As an example, a single instance of vital signs—heart rate, respiration, temperature, and blood pressure—for a single patient can be considered a set of data. A serial set of vital signs taken over time, placed into a context, and compared is considered information. For example, a dropping blood pressure, increasing heart rate, respiratory rate, and fever in an elderly, catheterized patient is recognized as being outside the norm for this type of patient. The recognition that this patient may be septic and needs certain nursing and medical interventions reflects information synthesis (knowledge) based on nursing knowledge and experience.

Figure 1 builds on the work of Graves and Corcoran by providing a depiction of the relationship of data, information, and knowledge. As data are transformed into information and information into knowledge, each level increases in complexity and requires greater application of human intellect. There are multiple feedback loops among the three concepts of data, information, and knowledge. The circles overlap purposefully because the precise distinction among these three concepts becomes blurred at their borders.

Data, which are processed to information and then knowledge, may be obtained from individuals, families, communities, and populations. Data, information, and knowledge are of concern to nurses in all areas of practice. For example, data derived from direct care of an individual patient are described in the previous scenario. Data may then be compiled across patients and aggregated for decision-making by nurse administrators. Further aggregation may address communities and populations. Nurse-educators may create case studies using these data, and nurse-researchers may access aggregated data for systematic study.

The concepts of nursing data, information, and knowledge resonated with informatics nurse specialists and others in the nursing community. The Graves and Corcoran (1989) work was widely cited by others.

Figure 1. Transformation of Data to Knowledge.

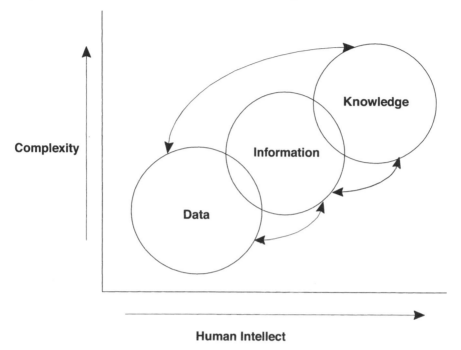

In a later work, the concepts of data, information, and knowledge are more clearly identified as a conceptual framework for the study of NI (Graves et al., 1995). Applying more current terminology, the Graves and Corcoran elements of data, information, and knowledge are part of the metastructure of nursing informatics, meaning that these elements are overarching concepts for the specialty of NI.

Nurses have been recognized as primary processors of information for over 30 years (Jydstrup and Gross, 1966; Zielstroff, 1981). In fact, Jydstrup and Gross estimated that nurses in acute care spent 30% to 40% of their time in information processing activities in the 1960s. Given the significant increases in the rate of data and information generation, it is likely that nurses currently spend even more time managing information.

In more recent years, the concept of nurses as information managers has been expanded to the idea that nurses are knowledge workers. *Knowledge work* is described by Drucker (1993) as nonrepetitive, nonroutine work consuming considerable levels of cognitive activity.

Knowledge workers use analytical and theoretical knowledge in sophisticated ways and develop complex manual skills. Thus, knowledge workers are often specialists. Business literature discusses knowledge as the basic means of production in contemporary organizations and that organizations are staffed by teams of knowledge workers (Drucker, 1993). Sorrells-Jones and Weaver (1999) state that these concepts are not yet widespread within health care, but clearly nurses and other providers fit the definition of a knowledge worker.

Nurse knowledge workers require support from informatics solutions for at least these processes: (a) storing clinical data, (b) translating clinical data to information, (c) linking clinical data and domain knowledge, and (d) aggregating clinical data (Snyder-Halpern, Corcoran-Perry, and Narayan, 2001). Currently, informatics solutions better support the first two processes. Therefore, it is critical that NI attends to the needs of nurses as knowledge workers by optimizing information technology support for all four processes.

Sciences Underpinning Nursing Informatics

The second contribution of Graves and Corcoran (1989) is a definition of nursing informatics (NI) that has been widely accepted in the field. It states that NI is a combination of nursing science, information science, and computer science to manage and process nursing data, information, and knowledge to facilitate the delivery of health care. Their central notion is that the application of these three core sciences—information science, computer science, and nursing science—is what makes NI unique and differentiates it from other informatics specialties.

In addition to these three core sciences, other sciences may be required to solve informatics issues. For instance, if an informatics nurse specialist is interested in the support of clinical decision-making, then cognitive science may be crucial to weave in with the core sciences. On the other hand, if the informatics nurse specialist is dealing with a system's implementation in an institution, an understanding of organizational theory may be much more pertinent to include in the informaticist's repertoire. Likewise, those studying nursing vocabularies would be wise to have a full understanding of linguistics. Because each informatics nurse specialist must tailor the theoretical support to their area of interest or subspecialty, many sciences may be appropriate to add to the core of information, computer, and nursing sciences.

Although the core sciences underpin the work in NI, the practice of the specialty is considered an applied rather than a basic science. The combination of sciences creates a unique blend that is greater than just the sum of its parts, a unique combination that creates the definitive specialty of NI. Further, informatics realizes its full potential within health care when it is grounded within a discipline; in this case, nursing. Computer and information science alone do little if they are not applied to a discipline. Through application, informatics can solve critical information management issues of concern to a discipline.

Concepts and Tools from Information Science and Computer Science

Informatics tools and methods from computer and information sciences are considered fundamental elements of nursing informatics (NI), including:

- Information technology

- Information structures

- Information management and communication

Information technology includes computer hardware, software, communication, and network technologies, which are derived primarily from computer science. The other two concepts are derived primarily from information science. First, *information structures* organize data, information, and knowledge for processing by computers. Second, *information management and communication* is an elemental process within informatics. This basic process is facilitated by information technology that distinguishes informatics from more traditional methods of information management. Thus, NI incorporates three more concepts: information technology, information structures, and the management and communication of information. Underpinning all of these are human–computer interaction concepts.

Human–Computer Interaction and Ergonomics Concepts

Human–computer interaction (HCI) and ergonomics concepts are fundamental concerns for the informatics nurse specialist. Essentially, HCI deals with people and computers and the ways they influence each other (Dix et al., 1998). This area blends psychology and/or cognitive science, applied work in computer science (Patel and Kaufman, 1998), sociology, and information science into the design, development, purchase, implementation, and evaluation of applications. For example, an informatics nurse specialist would assess an application before purchase to see if the application design complements the way nurses cognitively process a medication order. A related concept is usability or specific issues of human performance during computer interactions within a particular context (Rubin, 1994). Usability issues address the efficiency and effectiveness of an application (e.g., the ease of learning an application, the ease of using an application, or the speed and errors committed during application use) (Staggers, In press).

The term *ergonomics* is typically used in the United States to focus on the design and implementation of equipment, tools, and machines related to human safety, comfort, and convenience (Langendoen and Costa, 1994). In computing environments, ergonomics concepts commonly refer to attributes of physical equipment, and might be used to optimally arrange workstations and chairs to promote work in an intensive care unit, for example.

HCI, usability, and ergonomics are related concepts. All have as their goal the design of information, information technology, and equipment to promote optimal task completion. Although health care has been slow to embrace the use of HCI concepts, these concepts are essential for creating, selecting, implementing, and evaluating information structures and information technology of use to nurses and patients. Because of their fundamental nature, HCI concepts are listed as a NI assumption and an overarching standard for NI performance later in this document.

Phenomena of Nursing

The phenomena of nursing are the nurse, patient, health, and environment. Actions within nursing are based on the decisions made about these four phenomena. *Decision-making* is the process of choosing among alternatives. The decisions that nurses make can be characterized by both the quality of decisions that must be made and the impact of the actions resulting from those decisions. As knowledge workers, nurses make numerous decisions that affect the life and well-being of individuals, families, and communities. The process of decision-making in nursing is guided by the concept of critical thinking. *Critical thinking* is the intellectually disciplined process of actively and skillfully using knowledge to conceptualize, apply, analyze, synthesize, and/or evaluate data and information as a guide to belief and action (Scriven and Paul, 1997).

Nurses' decision-making includes behaviors, as well as cognitive processes, in an array of decisions, usually surrounding a cluster of issues rather than single decisions. For example, nurses use data transformed into information to determine interventions for patients, families, communities, and populations. Nurses make decisions about potential patient problems and preventive recommendations. They also make decisions based on inter-relationships with others (such as patients, physicians, or social workers) and decisions within specific environments (such as executive offices, classrooms, and research laboratories). In summary, the elements of interest for NI are:

- Data, information, and knowledge

- Nursing science, information science, and computer science

- Nurse, patient, health, and environment

- Decision-making

- Information structures; managing and communicating information and information technology

Terms and Definitions

Although well-established, nursing informatics (NI) is an evolving field that will continue to change rapidly. Definitions and theoretical structures for the specialty have been proposed, but they can be expected to continue to develop over time before stable concepts and definitions are realized.

Terms Used to Label the Role of the Nurse in Informatics

Various terms are in use describing the role of the registered nurse who practices informatics. They include:

- Nurse informaticist

- Informatics nurse

- Informatics nurse specialist

- Clinical informaticist

- Informaticist

In this document, the term informatics nurse specialist (INS) is used to encompass all these terms.

The informatics nurse specialist is a registered nurse who is educationally prepared at least at the master's degree level, preferably within nursing. This nurse's graduate level preparation is distinguished by a depth of knowledge of informatics and nursing theory and practice, validated experience in informatics practice, and competence in advanced informatics skills.

Evolution of the Definition of Nursing Informatics

A myriad of definitions have been proposed for nursing informatics (NI) in the past as discussed in Staggers and Thompson (In review). They may be categorized into three areas:

- Technology-focused definitions

- Conceptually focused definitions, and

- Role-oriented definitions

Technology-focused definitions

A definition for NI appeared as early as 1980. Scholes and Barber (1980, p. 70) stated that NI is, "The application of computer technology to all fields of nursing—nursing service, nurse education, and nursing research." Ball and Hannah (1984) modified an early definition of medical informatics, acknowledging that all health care professionals are part of medical informatics. Therefore, NI was defined as "those collected informational technologies which concern themselves with the patient care decision-making process performed by health care practitioners" (p. 3). A year later, Hannah (1985, p. 181) continued the emphasis on technology and added the concept of role within NI in the following definition:

> The use of information technologies in relation to those functions within the purview of nursing, and that are carried out

by nurses when performing their duties. Therefore, any use of information technologies by nurses in relation to the care of their patients, the administration of health care facilities, or the educational preparation of individuals to practice the discipline is considered nursing informatics.

Saba and McCormick (1986) did not specifically use the term NI in their first book, but organized book chapters around computer applications in the four areas of nursing. They defined nursing information systems as systems that use computers to process nursing data into information to support all types of nursing activities or functions.

The emphasis on technology is not limited to early definitions. Zielstorff et al. (1990) also support technology's significance in NI. More recently, Hannah (Hannah, Ball, and Edwards, 1994) and Saba and McCormick (1996) continue to stress the role of technology in NI as it supports the functions of nursing. Hannah et al. continued with her original definition for NI, and Saba and McCormick (1996, p. 226) provided this newer definition:

> The use of technology and/or a computer system to collect, store, process, display, retrieve, and communicate timely data and information in and across health care facilities that administer nursing services and resources, manage the delivery of patient and nursing care, link research resources and findings to nursing practice, and apply educational resources to nursing education.

These authors make a salient point about the principal role technology can play in informatics. In fact, for some practitioners, technology is the dominant issue. For others, NI is defined from a more conceptual view.

Conceptually focused definitions

Conceptual approaches to the emerging NI specialty began in the mid-1980s. These approaches gained acceptance in the 1990s.

Schwirian—Schwirian (1986), in a less frequently cited paper, stressed the need for a "solid foundation of NI knowledge, [that] should have focus, direction, and cumulative properties" (p. 134). She emphasized the need for research to be "proactive and model driven rather than reactive and problem-driven" (p. 134). Schwirian cited Hannah's (1985) more technology-oriented definition of NI, but produced a model that expanded thinking beyond just a focus on technology. Her research model outlined a pyramid of users, nursing-related information, goals, and computers (hardware and software) interconnected with bidirectional arrows. Nursing informatics activity lies within the intersection of the other elements. Meant as a stimulus for research in NI, the model could have been used to guide thinking about NI practice as well. The model depicts the inter-relationships among components and includes new concepts of nursing-related information, goals, and context.

Grobe—In 1988, Grobe described nursing informatics as ". . . the application of the principles of information science and theory to the study, scientific analysis, and management of nursing information for purposes of establishing a body of nursing knowledge" (p. 29). This definition was developed by an international team of nurses in the International Medical Informatics Association (IMIA). The timing of the release of this definition may have hindered its adoption because Graves and Corcoran released a paper about the scope of NI shortly thereafter.

Graves and Corcoran—Graves and Corcoran (1989) provided the first widely cited definition of NI, which downplayed the role of technology and incorporated a more conceptually oriented viewpoint:

> A combination of computer science, information science, and nursing science designed to assist in the management and processing of nursing data, information, and knowledge to support the practice of nursing and the delivery of nursing care (p. 227).

This definition broadened the horizon beyond technology. It also provided the first acknowledgment of an information–knowledge link. Graves and Corcoran's definition allowed a concentration on the purpose of technology rather than technology itself. Their transformation of the definition for NI changed the focus from technology to information concepts by expressly incorporating information science as part of the theoretical basis for NI. The centrality of nursing practice in the Graves and Corcoran definition also helps to support the need for NI as a distinct specialty within health informatics.

The 1989 definition was abstracted from earlier work by Graves and Corcoran (1988). The earlier paper placed the concepts of nursing data, decisions, and processes within a theoretical model showing the flow of data, information, and knowledge and the relationships among these key nursing processes. The model described how both research and clinical decision-making impact patient care and serve to build domain knowledge. After identifying the "flow of symbolic content in the discipline of nursing" (p. 172), Graves and Corcoran identified how information system technology could be used to facilitate each of the identified processes and transformations. Interestingly, in the 1989 work the authors removed the context of nursing and de-emphasized the interrelationships among technology, nurse, and patients from their broader model developed in a previous paper. Fewer nurses recognize the fundamental contribution of the earlier paper, as evidenced by the more frequent citation of the 1989 paper (Staggers and Thompson, In review).

Turley—Turley (1996) presents one of the more recent efforts at describing NI. He identified three themes for NI definitions and then proposed a new NI model. Although he analyzed previous definitions of NI, he did not propose a new definition for the field. By focusing on model development, his paper continued a conceptual approach to informatics. Turley's major contribution was adding cognitive science to a model comprised of the original three sciences proposed by Graves and Corcoran (1989). Turley acknowledged the growing interdisciplinary nature of health care and also focused on nursing's unique contributions to informatics.

Role-oriented definitions

At the time of the Graves and Corcoran paper (1989), informatics nurse specialists were becoming more prevalent. The early technology-related definitions suited these individuals because they emphasized the technological aspect of nurses' roles. As NI gained recognition as a nursing specialty, the ANA's Council on Computer

Applications in Nursing (ANA, 1992) provided a new definition for the field. The ANA expanded on the work of others by incorporating the role of the informatics nurse specialist into Graves and Corcoran's earlier definition:

> A specialty that integrates nursing science, computer science, and information science in identifying, collecting, processing, and managing data and information to support nursing practice, administration, education and research; and to expand nursing knowledge. The purpose of nursing informatics is to analyze information requirements; design, implement and evaluate information systems and data structures that support nursing; and identify and apply computer technologies for nursing (ANA, 1992).

The concepts of the systems life cycle first appeared in this definition. Unfortunately, this definition has not been frequently cited in subsequent work (e.g., Henry, 1995; Saba and McCormick, 1996; Turley, 1996).

In 1994, ANA modified its definition in an effort to legitimize the specialty and to guide efforts to create a certification exam. Although the 1994 (ANA) definition continues to provide information on the role of the informatics nurse specialist, the concepts from the systems life cycle are replaced with a more generic discussion of the NI role.

> Nursing informatics is the specialty that integrates nursing science, computer science, and information science in identifying, collecting, processing, and managing data and information to support nursing practice, administration, education, research, and expansion of nursing knowledge. Nursing informatics supports the practice of all nursing specialties, in all sites and settings whether at the basic or advanced level. The practice includes the development of applications, tools, processes, and structures that assist nurses with the management of data in taking care of patients or in supporting their practice of nursing (p. 3).

Although work on NI definitions within the international arena has occurred, this document concentrates on the NI definitions for North America. Given the relative newness of the NI specialty, having independent thought about definitions is healthy. Then, in the future, international consensus about definitions could occur.

A New Definition for Nursing Informatics

A new definition is needed to address the core elements identified—nurse, patient, health, environment, decision-making and nursing data, information, knowledge, information structures, and information technology. The construct of health is considered to be ubiquitous within nursing, environment, and patients; therefore, this concept is not reiterated within the new definition. Previous definitions underemphasize the role of the patient in informatics, do not mention information communication, and only imply that data and information are used in nurses' decision-making. In particular, the role of patients has dramatically changed in recent years as patients access and evaluate their own health information and become more participative in their own health care decision-making. Recently, nurses have assumed new roles as information brokers and information interpreters.

New Definition for Nursing Informatics

Nursing informatics is a specialty that integrates nursing science, computer science, and information science to manage and communicate data, information, and knowledge in nursing practice. Nursing informatics facilitates the integration of data, information, and knowledge to support patients, nurses, and other providers in their decision-making in all roles and settings. This support is accomplished through the use of information structures, information processes, and information technology.

The Goal of Nursing Informatics

The goal of nursing informatics (NI) is to improve the health of populations, communities, families, and individuals by optimizing information management and communication. This includes the use of technology in the direct provision of care, establishing effective administrative systems, managing and delivering educational experiences, supporting life-long learning, and supporting nursing research.

The Role of the Informatics Nurse Specialist

There are many activities inherent in the role of informatics nurse specialists (Willson, et al., 2000). These nurses typically concentrate on a subset of possible activities. Role activities include, but are not limited to, the following:

- Employ the information systems life cycle and other tools and processes to analyze data, information and information system requirements.

- Design, develop, select, and evaluate information technology, data structures, and decision-support mechanisms into an integrated information system. These systems support patients, nurses and their information management and human-computer interactions within health care contexts.

- Facilitate the creation of nursing knowledge.

In part because of the strong influence that emerging technology has in supporting the work of the informatics nurse specialist, the role is continually evolving. However, the following general roles are identified: project manager, consultant, educator, researcher, product developer, decision support/outcomes manager, and advocate/policy developer. The concept of the informatics nurse specialist as a change agent practicing in interdisciplinary environments is common to all roles.

Project Manager

In the project management role, informatics nurse specialists perform activities that implement the systems life cycle, including: analyzing, designing, developing, selecting, testing, implementing, and evaluating new or modified informatics solutions and data structures that support nursing and the delivery of patient care. The informatics nurse specialist is a catalyst for developing and revising policies and procedures based on system design, workflow reengineering, and input from system users. The project management role combines the skills of communication, change management, process analysis, risk assessment, scope definition, and team building, in conjunction with business and application knowledge in the management of projects involving informatics solutions. Informatics nurse specialists in this role provide input to the organization's strategic plan, evaluate the effectiveness of their projects, and continually strive to improve the quality and efficiency of their informatics solutions.

Consultant

Informatics nurse specialists in the consultant role apply their informatics knowledge and skills to serve as a resource to clients both formally and informally, in external and internal settings. Flexibility, good communication skills, breadth and depth of clinical and informatics knowledge, and excellent interpersonal skills are needed to respond to what can be rapidly changing projects and demands. This diverse role may involve assisting individuals and groups in defining health care information problems and identifying methodologies for implementing, utilizing, and modifying informatics solutions and data structures that support health care access, delivery, and evaluation. A consultant might serve as the project manager for an informatics-related project or may assist the organization's project manager. Consultants may assist clients in writing requests for proposals (RFPs) to elicit vendor bids for informatics solutions and evaluating responses. Other activities may include, but are not limited to, process redesign, strategic/information technology (IT) planning, system implementation, writing informatics publications, reviewing clinical software products, performing market research, and assisting in the planning of conferences, academic, and professional development programs. Nursing informatics consultants may work for a consulting firm, be employed as staff of the organization where they consult, or have an independent consulting practice.

Educator

Education and training are critical components of many nursing informatics (NI) roles and activities, and may directly impact the success or failure of any new/modified informatics solution. Teaching nurses, nursing students, patients, health care consumers, and others about the effective and ethical uses of information technology, as well as NI concepts and theories, is essential for encouraging the optimal use of informatics solutions in nursing practice. Informatics nurse specialists in the educator role develop, implement, and evaluate NI curriculum and educational technologies that meet the educational needs of learners. In this role, educators assess and evaluate NI skills and competencies while providing feedback to learners regarding the effectiveness of the learning activity and the learner's ability to demonstrate newly acquired skills. Educators manage, evaluate, report, and utilize data and information related to learners and the educational delivery system. These informatics nurse specialists are the innovators in defining and developing educational technologies, integrating the solutions into the educational and practice environments, and challenging the systems and organizations to consider and embrace innovative informatics processes and solutions.

Researcher

Informatics nurse specialists in the researcher role conduct the research that underlies the design, development, implementation, and impact of informatics solutions. This includes, but is not limited to:

- Basic research on symbolic representation of nursing phenomena
- Basic research on clinical decision-making in nursing
- Applied research in development of prototype systems
- Patients' use of information tools and resources for health information
- Effective methods for information systems implementation
- Human factors or ergonomics research about the design and impact of systems on patients, nurses, and their interactions
- Evaluation research on the effects of systems on the processes and outcomes of patient care
- Usability testing of applications

For example, conducting research to develop and refine standardized nursing languages is essential in defining, describing, and evaluating data, information, and knowledge relative to patient care. Other examples of NI research might include determining organizational attributes facilitating implementation success, investigating the impact and efficacy of hardware and software informatics solutions, linking nursing interventions to outcomes in large data sets, or determining effective nurse–patient interactions in telehealth contexts. Informatics nurse specialist researchers conduct research using systematic methods of inquiry, including traditional research techniques and newer techniques such as data mining or searching data in informatics solutions and data repositories.

Product Developer

Informatics nurse specialists are assuming expanded roles in the marketing, development, and support of systems software and hardware. In this role, informatics nurse specialists participate in the process of designing, developing, and marketing quality informatics solutions for nurses. Understanding the information needs of nurses, nursing, and patient care, as well as knowledge of business, client services, projected market directions, product design, product development methods, market research, contemporary programming, and modeling language are essential for practicing in a product development role.

Decision Support/Outcomes Manager

As aggregate data are made available from systems, they are used by informatics nurse specialists in a decision support/outcomes management role. Outcomes may be related to any area of nursing practice—clinical, education, research, or administration. For example, outcomes may be determined for patients, families, populations, and institutions. Nurses in this role use system tools to maintain data integrity and reliability, facilitate data aggregation and analysis, identify outcomes, and develop performance measurements. Performing in this role enables nurses to contribute to the development of a knowledge base consisting of the data, information, theories, and models that are used by nurses in decision-making and managing nursing-related problems.

Advocate/Policy Developer

The role of the informatics nurse specialist in advocacy and health policy development continues to expand. Informatics nurse specialists are key to infrastructure development of health policy; that is, knowing the data and information content, the structure of data, and the informatics solutions with those attributes. Informatics nurse specialists are experts in defining the data needed and the structure, management, and availability of those data for decision-making, and as such they advocate for patients, clients, providers, and the enterprise. Policy development may be at any level—a work center, institution, state, national, or international. Role activities include advocating for the ethical use of data and information, evaluating, developing, writing, and implementing policies. Regardless of the level or activity, informatics nurse specialists are active partners in the development of health policy, particularly related to information management and communication, confidentiality and security, patient safety, infrastructure development, and economics.

Other Roles of the Informatics Nurse Specialist

New roles for the informatics nurse specialist have emerged. For example, informatics nurse specialists may be entrepreneurs developing products, relevant content, or the user interface for consumer informatics (Web sites). Other roles may include executive-level positions such as chief information officer (CIO) in provider and vendor organizations, managing an independent practice, or owning a business as a health database designer. Clearly, in the future new roles will continue to evolve.

Tenets of Nursing Informatics

- Nursing informatics is a distinct area of specialty practice within nursing. It has a unique body of knowledge, formal preparation within the specialty, and identifiable techniques and methods.

- Nursing informatics includes both a clinical practice and non-clinical area of practice.

- Nursing informatics supports the efforts of nurses to improve the quality of care and the welfare of health care consumer. Information or informatics methods alone do not improve patient care; rather, this information is used by clinicians and managers to effect improvements in care, information management and patient outcomes.

- Although concerned with information technology, nursing informatics focuses on delivering the right information to the right person at the right time.

- Human factors (human–computer interaction [HCI], ergonomics, and usability) concepts are interwoven throughout the practice of NI.

- Nursing informatics' key concerns include ensuring the confidentiality and security of health care data and information and advocating privacy.

- Nursing informatics promotes innovative, emerging, and established information technologies.

- Nursing informatics collaborates with and is closely linked to other health-related informatics specialties.

The Boundaries of Nursing Informatics

This section discusses what nursing informatics (NI) is and is not. It also summarizes the differences between NI and other specialties in nursing. To reiterate, nursing informatics is a specialty that integrates nursing science, computer science, and information science to manage and communicate data, information, and knowledge in nursing practice. Nursing informatics facilitates the integration of data, information, and knowledge to support patients, nurses, and other providers in their decision-making in all roles and settings. This support is accomplished through the use of information structures and information technology.

Nursing Informatics Differentiated From Other Nursing Specialties

The difference between NI and other nursing specialties is the melding of informatics concepts, tools, and methods with nursing. It is the integration of informatics tools and methods, such as information structure, information technology, and information management and communication that distinguish NI. However, we should not confuse what computers can do with the essence of the work at hand. The work of nursing is at the heart of NI and informatics tools and methods only facilitate this work.

Although some outside the specialty might consider NI synonymous with information technology, focusing on technology alone does not define NI. Whereas information technology is used extensively within the specialty, information technology is a tool to support the principal concern of NI: nursing information management and communication. Thus, the data and information are central to NI; information technology assists in the optimal management and communication of nursing information.

Information is central to the practice of nursing and all nurses must be skilled in managing and communicating information. However, nurses outside NI are primarily concerned with the *content* of that information, whereas informatics nurse specialists focus on the design, structure, and presentation of information and how these issues impact nurses' decision-making. Table 1 distinguishes the foci of nursing and NI.

Informatics Competencies

Although this document focuses on the informatics nurse specialist, informatics competencies are needed by all nurses whether or not they specialize in nursing informatics. As nursing settings become ubiquitous computing environments, all nurses must be both information and computer literate. Competencies are described for two levels of nurses not schooled in informatics (beginning and experienced nurse) and a third level for the nurse prepared in informatics (Staggers, Gassert, and Curran, 2001). The scope and depth of knowledge in informatics increases with each level from beginning nurse to informatics nurse specialist. Also, each level of competency builds on the previous one. Therefore, before becoming an informatics nurse specialist, the nurse is expected to have demonstrated proficiency in the competencies outlined in the beginning and experienced nurse competency levels. Informatics competencies for nurses may be organized into computer skills, information literacy skills, and overall informatics competencies.

Beginning Nurse

The beginning nurse is a nurse preparing for initial entry into nursing practice or who has just begun a nursing career. This nurse is

Table 1. Comparison of Metastructures, Concepts, and Tools of Nursing and Nursing Informatics

Nursing Focus	Nursing Informatics Focus
Nurses, patients, health, environment	Nursing data, information, and knowledge
Content of information	Design, structure, and presentation of information as it impacts nurses' decision-making
Using information applications and technology	Optimizing information structures, applications, and technology for use in managing and communicating data, information, and knowledge

expected to have fundamental information management and computer literacy skills. Beginning nurses use existing informatics solutions and available information to manage their practice.

Computer literacy skills

Computer literacy is a set of skills that allow individuals to use computer technology to accomplish tasks. These include, but are not limited to, basic computer technology skills such as using a word processor, database, spreadsheet, or using applications to document patient care or communicate via e-mail. These skills are necessary for all nurses, but not sufficient for informatics nurse specialists. Thus, a nurse who takes classes focused on learning applications such as word processing or presentation graphics may be considered computer literate, but is not an informatics nurse specialist.

Information literacy skills

Information literacy is a set of abilities allowing individuals to recognize when information is needed and to locate, evaluate, and use that information appropriately (Association of Colleges and Research Libraries [ACRL], 2000). The primary focus of information literacy is on information access and evaluation. Examples are performing bibliographic retrieval and retrieving and evaluating information from Internet sources. These relevant skills are primarily derived from library science. According to the ACRL, an information literate individual is able to:

- Determine the extent of information needed.

- Access the needed information effectively and efficiently.

- Evaluate information and its sources critically.

- Incorporate selected information into one's knowledge base.

- Use information effectively to accomplish a specific purpose.

- Understand the economic, legal, and social issues surrounding the use of information, and access and use information ethically and legally (ACRL, 2000, p. 2).

Overall informatics competencies

The following overall informatics competencies are required of beginning nurses, those individuals first learning about or entering into nursing practice. Overall informatics activities may include but are not limited to:

- Identifying, collecting, and recording data relevant to the nursing care of patients.

- Analyzing and interpreting patient and nursing information as part of the planning for the provision of nursing services.

- Using informatics applications designed for the practice of nursing.

- Implementing public and institutional policies related to privacy, confidentiality, and security of information. These include patient care information, confidential employer information, and other information gained in the nurse's professional capacity.

Experienced Nurse

Experienced nurses have proficiency in one or more domains of interest. This nurse is highly skilled in information management and communication. Experienced nurses have information and computer literacy skills to support their major area of practice. These nurses see relationships among data elements, and make judgments based on trends and patterns within these data. Experienced nurses use current informatics solutions, but also collaborate with the informatics nurse specialist to suggest improvements to these informatics solutions (Staggers, Gassert, and Curran, 2001). In addition to competencies for beginning nurses, experienced nurse activities include at least the following:

- Use system applications to manage data, information, and knowledge within their specialty area.

- Participate as a content expert to evaluate information and assist others in developing information structures and systems to support their area of nursing practice.

- Promote the integrity of and access to information to include, but not limited to, confidentiality, legal, ethical, and security issues.

- Being actively involved in efforts to improve information management and communication (e.g., supports the development and use of standardized nursing languages).

- Act as an advocate or leader for incorporating innovations and informatics concepts into their area of specialty.

Informatics Nurse Specialist

The informatics nurse specialist is expected to have the competencies outlined in the beginning and experienced nurse competency levels. Moving beyond computer skills, information literacy skills, and overall informatics competencies, the informatics nurse specialist demonstrates the competencies reflected in the standards of practice and professional performance.

The Interdisciplinary Nature of Nursing Informatics

Nursing informatics is a practice specialty and an applied science. Informatics nurse specialists frequently collaborate with other informaticists to optimize nursing information management and communication. To effect information management and communication, NI may use concepts from many sources besides the three core sciences, which may include, but are not limited to, linguistics, cognitive science, engineering, managerial science, and educational theories.

The practice of NI can be, and often is, within interdisciplinary environments. In fact, most informatics nurse specialists function in interdisciplinary environments, working collaboratively with others in team-oriented or patient-centered work processes. However, the central issues of concern to the specialty of NI are embedded within the discipline itself—data, information, and knowledge used for nurses' decision-making in any environment, in any nursing specialty. Although the work of informatics nurse specialists is typically within interdisciplinary teams, informatics nurse specialists add a nursing voice to these interdisciplinary environments and often ensure that nurses' requirements are adequately addressed within these contexts.

The difference between NI and other informatics specialties rests with NI's focus on the information management and communication of nursing data, information, and knowledge. NI has many elements in common with other informatics specialties; for example, informatics tools methods and concepts from information and computer science. Therefore, the boundaries between nursing informatics and other informatics specialties are not rigid, but dynamic and fluid, allowing for information processing to occur beyond just this one informatics specialty.

Ethics in Nursing Informatics

Nursing's long history includes primary concern for the patient or client and commitment to the professional code of ethics for nurses. Therefore, the *Code of Ethics for Nurses* (ANA, 2001) serves as a framework for the informatics nurse specialist who faces ethical issues and ethical dilemmas. This concern for both the patient and commitment to the Code form the foundation for the informatics nurse specialist's unique expertise and insight in this area.

Although the informatics nurse specialist may not be functioning as a clinician, the issues of confidentiality, security, and privacy surrounding the patient, clinician, and enterprise and the associated data, information, and knowledge are of paramount concern. These issues provide significant opportunities to the information nurse specialist for ethical analysis, decision-making, and subsequent action. For example, the explosion of the human genetic mapping and testing technologies is creating valuable new insights into disease identification and treatment opportunities. However, this also produces potentially damaging outcomes if that same information is incorrectly reported or inadequately safeguarded and becomes available to the wrong person or agency. The informatics nurse specialist in this environment has a responsibility to advocate for confidentiality, data integrity and security, quality management of information, and appropriate decision-making.

More powerful information technologies permit new computing approaches and greater data aggregation and linkage capabilities. But as these opportunities expand, the correct application of the methodologies needs continuing evaluation and monitoring. To ensure that appropriate informatics solutions are implemented, the informatics nurse specialist is instrumental in posing questions, such as:

- Has informed consent of the health care consumer been adequately secured?

- Are the databases protected from external and internal compromise?

- Have the appropriate retention and disposition policies been established?

- Are data information management policies enforced?

- Can client anonymity be maintained?

- Are technical, consultant, and vendor personnel accountable for adherence to security and confidentiality mandates?

- Is the researcher accountable for adherence to security and confidentiality mandates?

- Does the Institutional Review Board (IRB) include examination of the information and database management strategies during the review process to ensure adequate protection of the individual subject, the researcher, and the organization?

Health care professionals are accustomed to adhering to a professional code of ethics. Others in the information management and information systems environments may not embrace such a tradition. Ethical questions or issues arise when common corporate business practices run counter to the ethical mandates of health care professionals. The informatics nurse specialist brings an integrated, systems perspective to discussions of the ethical issues posed by such questions as:

- Is a code of ethics integrated into the expanding distributed environment of Internet health information and health care service delivery?

- What standards are in place to address concerns about conflict of interest when health information resources are posted as part of an organization's or company's marketing strategy?

- Is the individual responding to the e-mail or Internet site query truly a qualified clinician appropriately licensed to practice?

- Are appropriate safeguards in place to protect the sender's identity and privacy, the content and integrity of messages, and the respondent's identity?

The Future of Nursing Informatics

After the Graves and Corcoran (1989) article, others proposed adding the concept of wisdom to the triad of data, information, and knowledge (Nelson and Joos, 1989). *Wisdom* may be defined as the appropriate use of data, information, and knowledge in making decisions and implementing nursing actions. It includes the ability to integrate data, information, and knowledge with professional values when managing specific human problems.

Some nursing informatics (NI) experts believe strongly that wisdom is the purview of humans and cannot or should not be considered as a function within technology. Others believe that informatics solutions consistent with professional values and useful to expert nurses will require the incorporation of wisdom. This controversy makes the inclusion of wisdom into the triad of data, information, and knowledge currently an unresolved issue within NI.

This document represents the state of nursing informatics. However, a number of trends in the field of informatics are currently evident and are mentioned here:

- Ubiquitous computing is becoming a reality and the continued innovation and miniaturization of technology is evident. Consequently, partnering between nurses in all specialties and new technologies is becoming imperative.

- Technological innovations are challenging many traditional processes within health care.

- Telecommunications technologies are one set of tools used in nursing practice.

- Core competencies across informatics specialties should be identified in the near future. Therefore, the distinctions among informatics specialties will continue to blur.

- The speed of information transfer and the increasing availability of communications technologies will impact nurses and informatics nurse specialists in the future, making nursing practice and NI, in particular, more international in practice with worldwide standards, competencies, and curricula.

This section outlined the scope of practice for informatics nurse specialists. In the next section, the standards of practice and professional performance for informatics nurse specialists are addressed.

INFORMATICS NURSE SPECIALIST
STANDARDS OF PRACTICE

Nursing informatics is the specialty that integrates nursing science, computer science, and information science to manage and communicate data, information, and knowledge in nursing practice. Nursing informatics facilitates the integration of data, information, and knowledge to support patients, nurses, and other providers in their decision-making in all roles and settings. This support is accomplished through the use of information structures, information processes, and information technology.

The goal of NI is to improve the health of populations, communities, families, and individuals by optimizing information management and communication. This includes the use of technology in the direct provision of care, in establishing effective administrative systems, in managing and delivering educational experiences, in supporting life-long learning, and in supporting nursing research.

The standards of practice for the informatics nurse specialist are organized around a general problem-solving framework that closely resembles the familiar nursing process of assessment, diagnosis, identification of outcomes, planning, implementation, and evaluation. The problem-solving framework supports all facets of informatics practice, including those without technology, and all areas of nursing practice. Informatics nurse specialists and other informaticians use a structured problem-solving method to identify and clarify issues and select, develop, implement, and evaluate informatics solutions. These steps are not mutually exclusive and topics may overlap multiple identified steps.

Informatics solution is a generic term used in this document to describe the product an informatics nurse specialist recommends after identifying and analyzing an issue. An informatics solution may encompass technology and nontechnology products such as developing a database, purchasing a new computer application, creating nursing vocabulary, designing informatics curricula, creating a spreadsheet, tailoring an application to a particular environment, designing a research study to describe required informatics competencies, describing information flow in a process redesign, or creating a structure for information presentation.

Several overarching standards inherent in every aspect of practice begin the discussion of the informatics nurse specialist standards of practice.

Overarching Standards of Practice for the Informatics Nurse Specialist

The informatics nurse specialist:

1. Incorporates theories, principles, and concepts from appropriate sciences into informatics practice. Examples of theories could include information, systems, and change theories. Principles and concepts could include project management, implementation methods, organizational culture, and database structures.

2. Integrates ergonomics and human–computer interaction (HCI) principles into informatics solution design, development, selection, implementation, and evaluation.

3. Systematically determines the social, legal, and ethical impact of an informatics solution within nursing and health care.

Standard I. Identify the Issue or Problem

The informatics nurse specialist synthesizes data, information, and knowledge to clarify informatics issues or problems.

Measurement Criteria

The informatics nurse specialist:

1. Conducts a needs assessment to refine the issue or problem.

   a. Analyzes current practice, workflow, and the potential impact of an informatics solution on that workflow.

   b. Involves crucial stakeholders in an issue or problem and its informatics solution.

c. Evaluates obtained information and findings for their pertinence to the informatics issue or problem.

d. Integrates current and future requirements into a vision for an informatics solution.

2. Incorporates principles and methods of recognized methodologies, such as structured systems analysis, into problem or issue identification.

3. Uses systematic methods to determine user and technical requirements for informatics issues.

4. Interprets the capabilities and limitations of legacy systems in integration planning and requirements determination.

5. Interprets current legislation, trends, and research affecting health information management.

6. Actively participates in strategic planning.

7. Conducts a market analysis for an informatics solution.

Standard II. Identify Alternatives

The informatics nurse specialist analyzes multiple approaches/solutions to the informatics issue or problem.

Measurement Criteria

The informatics nurse specialist:

1. Uses problem-solving tools and processes to identify and evaluate approaches and solutions to informatics issues and/or problems. These activities may include:

   a. Conducting a systems analysis to determine information needs.

   b. Developing functional and technical specifications based upon identified needs.

   c. Developing business process redesign recommendations.

   d. Analyzing costs and potential return on investment (ROI) as a basis for selecting and implementing informatics solutions.

e. Judging the fit of the proposed informatics solution with the strategic plan.

2. Uses analytical models to identify and evaluate approaches and solutions to informatics issues and/or problems. These activities may include:

   a. Developing conceptual, external, and internal models for representing information needs.

   b. Designing models of informatics solutions.

3. Prepares documents to describe information needs for the proposed informatics solution. These activities may include:

   a. Developing informal and formal requests for an informatics solution such as a request for information or an RFP.

   b. Preparing a response to a request for a proposed informatics solution.

   c. Using models to communicate to key stakeholders.

Standard III. Choose and Develop a Solution

The informatics nurse specialist develops an informatics solution for a specific issue or problem.

Measurement Criteria

The informatics nurse specialist:

1. Interprets capabilities and limitations of hardware and software and their relationship to the outcomes of proposed informatics solutions in health care.

2. Incorporates usability testing methods in choosing, developing and evaluating an informatics solution.

3. Analyzes economic, technical, and human resources available to support the informatics solution.

4. Incorporates established informatics standards into the informatics solution.

5. Selects an informatics solution by applying selection criteria appropriate for the targeted users and expected outcomes.

6. Develops an evaluation plan for the informatics solution including measurable outcomes and/or terminal objectives.

7. Develops an informatics solution such as designing a documentation tool, determining clinical vocabulary, tailoring an application to a specific environment, or writing a manuscript about an informatics topic.

8. Actively participates in contract development and negotiations, as appropriate.

Standard IV. Implement the Solution

The informatics nurse specialist manages the process for implementing the solution to the informatics issue or problem.

Measurement Criteria

The informatics nurse specialist:

1. Applies principles and concepts of project management to the implementation of the solution.

2. Demonstrates methods of effective project management when implementing the solution.

3. Demonstrates expertise as a project manager.

4. Designs strategies for effective funding of informatics solutions, which may include:

   a. Developing a budget plan for the procurement of resources and maintenance of an informatics solution.

   b. Determining priorities for requirements within budget constraints.

   c. Employing persuasive communication and political astuteness in funding strategies.

5. Develops policies, procedures, and guidelines based on research and analytical findings, which may include:

a. Supporting the implementation, use, and on-going maintenance of an informatics solution.

b. Ensuring the validity and integrity of data.

c. Promoting health and safety within the particular environment.

d. Ensuring the use of an effective informatics solution.

e. Ensuring the ethical use of informatics solution.

f. Ensuring the confidentiality and security of data and privacy for individuals.

6. Ensures that the informatics solution is in compliance with recognized standards from accrediting and regulatory agencies.

7. Manages strategies for implementing the informatics solution.

8. Applies performance or systems testing methodologies to all phases of implementation of the solution, which may include:

a. Developing procedures, policies, protocols, and scenarios for acceptance testing, conversions, and interface testing.

b. Developing a plan for testing implementation conversion and backup procedures.

c. Developing baseline criteria for system acceptance.

d. Recommending solutions for problems and impediments identified during performance/system testing.

9. Manages education activities for the informatics solution, which may include:

a. Developing an education plan based on measurable, learner-oriented outcomes.

b. Producing education materials based on educational principles.

c. Implementing educational activities for learners.

d. Using innovative educational techniques such as computer-based training or virtual reality as appropriate to learner populations and the specific informatics solution.

e. Evaluating all aspects of educational activities.

10. Applies knowledge of product design, information technologies, and client services to internal and external marketing activities to facilitate the adoption of the solution.

Standard V. Evaluate and Adjust Solutions

The informatics nurse specialist evaluates all processes and solutions used to address the informatics problem.

Measurement Criteria

The informatics nurse specialist:

1. Uses a variety of methods to evaluate the structure, process, and outcome of the informatics solution, which may include:

    a. Assessing the ROI.

    b. Conducting a benefits realization analysis at appropriate intervals during and after solution implementation.

    c. Using summative and formative techniques for a comprehensive evaluation approach.

    d. Using reliable and valid instruments to measure user satisfaction with the implemented informatics solution.

    e. Identifying the extent to which the project budget and schedule are met.

2. Analyzes the impact of the informatics solution on individuals, families, communities, and institutions affected by the solution, which may include:

    a. Adapting market analysis tools and techniques to identify recommended changes to the informatics solution.

    b. Using reliable and valid measures to analyze perceived and actual responses to the informatics solution.

    c. Creating written plans for ongoing analysis of the informatics solution's impact.

3. Disseminates results of evaluation to colleagues, stakeholders and others.

4. Reviews all prior steps in the problem-solving process and makes recommendations, which may include:

   a. Systematically assessing the quality and effectiveness of the problem-solving process and informatics solution.

   b. Using the results of the quality and effectiveness analysis to make or recommend process or structural changes.

   c. Incorporating the results of evaluations into policy, procedure, or protocol documentation.

   d. Changing educational programs based on findings.

5. Uses multiple methods, disseminates information and knowledge synthesized from evaluation activities.

INFORMATICS NURSE SPECIALIST STANDARDS OF PROFESSIONAL PERFORMANCE

Standard I. Quality of Nursing Informatics Practice

The informatics nurse specialist evaluates the quality and effectiveness of nursing informatics practice.

Measurement Criteria

The informatics nurse specialist:

1. Integrates knowledge of current professional practice standards, laws, and regulations into informatics practice.

2. Performs quality improvement activities, which may include:

    a. Identifying aspects of nursing informatics practice important for quality monitoring.

    b. Evaluating indicators used to monitor quality and effectiveness of nursing informatics practice.

    c. Collecting data to monitor quality and effectiveness of nursing informatics practice using structures developed for that purpose.

    d. Analyzing quality data to identify opportunities for improving nursing informatics practice.

    e. Formulating recommendations to improve nursing informatics practice or outcomes.

    f. Implementing activities to enhance the quality of nursing informatics practice.

    g. Developing, implementing, and evaluating policies and procedures to improve the quality of nursing informatics practice.

    h. Synthesizing information about the existing and emerging standards to apply to the nursing informatics practice.

3. Implements the results of quality activities to initiate changes in nursing informatics practice.

Standard II. Performance Appraisal

The informatics nurse specialist evaluates one's own nursing informatics practice in relation to professional practice standards and relevant statutes and regulations.

Measurement Criteria

The informatics nurse specialist:

1. Engages in and conducts performance appraisal on a regular basis, identifying areas of strengths as well as areas where professional development is needed.
2. Seeks constructive feedback regarding one's own practice.
3. Takes action to achieve goals identified during performance appraisal.
4. Seeks peer review as appropriate.

Standard III. Education

The informatics nurse specialist maintains knowledge and competency that reflects current nursing informatics (NI) practice.

Measurement Criteria

The informatics nurse specialist:

1. Maintains current skills and competencies.
2. Seeks new knowledge and skills appropriate to NI practice through professional development activities.
3. Seeks certification, if applicable.

Standard IV. Collegiality

The informatics nurse specialist contributes to the professional development of peers, informatics colleagues, and others.

Measurement Criteria

The informatics nurse specialist:

1. Shares knowledge and skills with peers and colleagues.

2. Contributes to informatics education of students, peers, and colleagues.

3. Provides constructive feedback regarding others' practice.

4. Promotes understanding and effective use of information management and information technology.

5. Promotes understanding of NI by translating NI concepts and practice to others.

6. Participates on multi-professional teams that evaluate health informatics practice.

7. Recommends changes in health care informatics using results from the evaluation of the quality and effectiveness of NI practice.

Standard V. Ethics

The informatics nurse specialist bases decisions and actions on ethical principles.

Measurement Criteria

The informatics nurse specialist:

1. Practices according to the current *Code of Ethics for Nurses* (ANA, 2001).

2. Develops methods to maintain confidentiality, and security of information, data, and knowledge.

3. Advocates for appropriate use of data, information, and knowledge.

4. Practices in a nonjudgmental and nondiscriminatory manner that is sensitive to human diversity.

5. Practices in a manner that preserves and protects human autonomy, dignity, and rights.

6. Seeks available resources as needed when formulating ethical decisions.

Standard VI. Collaboration

The informatics nurse specialist collaborates with others in the conduct of nursing informatics (NI) practice.

Measurement Criteria

The informatics nurse specialist:

1. Collaborates with patients and clients, families, informatics professionals, and others in informatics activities.

2. Collaborates with faculty in developing, maintaining, and evaluating educational and professional development informatics programs.

3. Collaborates with others in building the NI knowledge base. This may include activities such as publishing, policy development, and/or conducting research.

Standard VII. Research

The informatics nurse specialist contributes to the body of informatics knowledge.

Measurement Criteria

The informatics nurse specialist:

1. Integrates best available evidence into nursing informatics practice.

2. Conducts systematic inquiry of informatics problems and issues.

3. Disseminates information and knowledge related to systematic inquiry.

4. Develops informatics policies, procedures, and guidelines based on systematic inquiry.

5. Formulates an informatics research program.

Standards VIII. Resource Utilization

The informatics nurse specialist considers factors related to safety, effectiveness, cost, and impact in conducting informatics practice.

Measurement Criteria

The informatics nurse specialist:

1. Evaluates factors related to safety, effectiveness, costs, and impact when developing and implementing information management solutions.

2. Applies strategies to obtain appropriate resources for informatics initiatives.

3. Assigns tasks or delegates responsibilities appropriately based on the nursing informatics activity being conducted.

4. Promotes adoption of activities that assist others in becoming informed about costs, risks, and benefits of information management and information technology solutions.

Standard IX. Communication

The informatics nurse specialist employs effective communications.

Measurement Criteria

The informatics nurse specialist:

1. Is fluent in informatics terminology and standardized languages.

2. Articulates informatics requirements to other disciplines.

3. Interprets communication to and from others, such as informatics professionals, clinicians, patients, executives, and vendors.

4. Communicates complex concepts concisely.

5. Demonstrates persuasive abilities in communication.

6. Applies established guidelines to written communication.

GLOSSARY

Beginning nurse—A nurse preparing for initial entry into nursing practice or who has just begun a nursing career.

Data—Discrete entities that are described objectively without interpretation.

Experienced nurse—A nurse with proficiency in one or more domains of interest.

Informatics solution—A generic term used to describe the product an informatics nurse specialist recommends after identifying and analyzing an issue. Informatics solutions may encompass technology and nontechnology products such as information systems, new applications, nursing vocabulary, or informatics curricula.

Information—Data that are interpreted, organized, or structured.

Knowledge—Information that is synthesized so that relationships are identified and formalized.

Nursing informatics (NI)—A specialty that integrates nursing science, computer science, and information science to manage and communicate data, information, and knowledge in nursing practice. Nursing informatics facilitates the integration of data, information, and knowledge to support patients, nurses, and other providers in their decision-making in all roles and settings. This support is accomplished through the use of information structures, information processes, and information technology.

REFERENCES

American Nurses Association (ANA). (2001). *Code of Ethics for Nurses with Interpretive Statements*. Washington, DC: American Nurses Publishing.

―――. (1995). *Standards of Practice for Nursing Informatics*. Washington, DC: American Nurses Publishing.

―――. (1994). *Scope of Practice for Nursing Informatics*. Washington, DC: American Nurses Publishing.

―――. Council on Computer Applications in Nursing. (1992). *Report on the Designation of Nursing Informatics as a Nursing Specialty*. Congress of Nursing Practice unpublished report. Washington, DC: American Nurses Association.

The Association of Colleges and Research Libraries (ACRL). (2000). *Information Literacy Competency Standards for Higher Education*. San Antonio, TX: American Library Association.

Ball, M. J., and K. J. Hannah. (1984). *Using Computers in Nursing*. Reston, VA: Reston Publishing Co.

Blum, B. L. (1986) *Clinical Information Systems*, p. 35. New York: Springer-Verlag.

Brennan, P. F. (1994). The relevance of discipline. *Journal of the American Medical Informatics Association*, 1(2): 200–201.

Brennan, P. F., R. D. Zielstorff, J. G. Ozbolt, and I. Strombom. (1998). Setting a national research agenda in nursing informatics. In B. Cesnik, A. T. McCray, and J. R. Scherrer (eds). *Medinfo '98: Proceedings of the Ninth World Congress on Medical Informatics*, pp. 1188–1191. Amsterdam: IOS Press.

Dix, A., J. Finlay, G. Abowd, and R. Beale. (1998). *Human–Computer Interaction*. London: Prentice Hall Europe.

Drucker, P. F. (1993). *Post Capitalist Society*. New York: Harper Business Publishers.

Gassert, C. A. (2000). Academic preparation for nursing informatics. In Ball, M. J., K. J. Hannah, S. K. Newbold, and J. V. Douglas (eds). (2001). *Nursing Informatics: Where Caring and Technology Meet, 3rd ed.*, pp. 15–32. New York: Springer-Verlag.

Graves, J. R., L. K. Amos, S. Huether, L. Lange, and C. B. Thompson. (1995). Description of a graduate program in clinical nursing informatics. *Computers in Nursing* 13: 60–70.

Graves, J. R., and S. Corcoran. (1989). The study of nursing informatics. *Image* 21(4): 227–231.

———. (1988). Design of nursing information systems. *Journal of Professional Nursing* 4: 168–177.

Grobe, S. J. (1988). Nursing informatics competencies for nurse educators and researchers. In Peterson, H. E., and U. Gerdin-Jelger (eds). *Preparing Nurses for Using Information Systems: Recommended Informatics Competencies*, pp. 25–33. New York: National League for Nursing.

Hannah, K. J. (1985). Current trends in nursing in informatics: Implications for curriculum planning. In Hannah, K. J., E. J. Guillemin, and D. N. Conklin (eds). *Nursing Uses of Computers and Information Science*, pp. 181–187. Amsterdam: North-Holland.

Hannah, K. J., M. J. Ball, and M. J. A. Edwards. (1994). *Introduction to Nursing Informatics*. New York: Springer-Verlag.

Henry, S. (1995). Nursing informatics: State of the science. *Journal of Advanced Nursing* 22: 1182–1192.

Jydstrup, R. A., and J. J. Gross. (1966). Cost of information handling in hospitals. *Health Services Research* 1(3): 235–271.

Lange, L. L. (1997). Informatics nurse specialist: Roles in health care organizations. *Nursing Administration Quarterly* 21(3): 1–10.

Langendoen, D., and D. Costa. (1994). *The Home Office Computer Handbook*. New York: Windcrest/McGraw-Hill.

National Advisory Council on Nurse Education and Practice (NACNEP). (1997). *A National Agenda for Nursing Education and Practice*. Rockville, MD: U.S. Department of Health and Human Services, Health Resources and Services Administration.

National Center for Nursing Research (NCNR). (1993). *Nursing Informatics: Enhancing Patient Care: A Report of the NCNR Priority Expert Panel on Nursing Informatics/National Center for Nursing Research*, pp. 3–9. NIH Publication No. 93-2419. Bethesda, MD: U.S. Department of Health and Human Services.

Nelson, R., and I. Joos. (1989). On language in nursing: From data to wisdom. *PLN Vision* Fall: 6.

Panniers, T. L., and C. A. Gassert. (1996). Standards of practice and preparation for certification. In Mills, M. E., C. A. Romano, and B. R. Heller (eds). *Information Management in Nursing and Health Care*, pp. 280–287. Springhouse, PA: Springhouse Corporation.

Patel, V., and D. Kaufman. (1998). Medical informatics and the science of cognition. *Journal of the American Medical Informatics Association* 5(6): 493–502.

Rubin, J. (1994). *Handbook of Usability Testing: How to Plan, Design, and Conduct Effective Tests*. New York: John Wiley and Sons.

Saba, V. K., and K. A. McCormick. (1996). Nursing informatics. In *Essentials of Computers for Nurses, 2nd ed.* pp. 221–263. New York: McGraw-Hill.

———. (1986). *Essentials of Computers for Nurses*. Philadelphia: J. B. Lippincott.

Scholes, M., and B. Barber. (1980). Towards nursing informatics. In Linberg, D. A. D., and S. Kaihara (eds). *MEDINFO: 1980*, pp. 70–73. Amsterdam Netherlands: North-Holland.

Schwirian, P. (1986). The NI pyramid-A model for research in nursing informatics. *Computers in Nursing* 4(3): 134–136.

Scriven, M., and R. Paul. (1997). A working definition of critical thinking by Michael Scriven and Richard Paul. Available from http://lonestar.texas.net/~mseifert/crit2.html (from the Palo Alto College Critical Thinking Resource Home Page). Accessed September 18, 2001.

Snyder-Halpern, R., S. Corcoran-Perry, and S. Narayan. (2001). Developing clinical practice environments supportive of the knowledge work of nurses. *Computers in Nursing* 19(1): 17–23.

Sorrells-Jones, Jean, and Diana Weaver. (1999.) Knowledge workers and knowledge-intense organizations. Part 1: A. Promising framework for nursing and healthcare. *Journal of Nursing Administration* Jul/Aug; 29(7/8): 12–18.

Staggers, N. (In press). Human-computer interaction in health care organizations. In Englebardt, S., and R. Nelson. *Health Care Informatics: An Interdisciplinary Approach*. St. Louis, MO: Harcourt.

Staggers, N., and C. B. Thompson. (In review). The evolution of definitions for nursing informatics. *Journal of the American Medical Informatics Association*.

Staggers, N., C. A. Gassert, and C. Curran. (2001). Informatics competencies for nurses at four levels of practice. *Journal of Nursing Education* 40(7): 303–316.

Styles, M. M. (1989). *On Specialization in Nursing: Toward a New Empowerment*. Kansas City, MO: American Nurses Foundation.

Turley, J. (1996). Toward a model for nursing informatics. *Image* 28: 309–313.

Wilson, D., G. Bjornstad, et al. (2000) Nursing informatics career opportunities. In Carty, B. (ed). *Nursing Informatics: Education for Practice*. New York: Springer.

Zielstorff, R. (1981). How computer systems influence nursing activities in hospitals. In *The Proceedings of the First National Conference: Computer Technology and Nursing*, pp. 1–6. Bethesda, MD: National Institutes of Health.

Zielstorff, R., L. Abraham, H. Werley, V. K. Saba, and P. Schwirian. (1990). Guidelines for adopting innovations in computer-based information systems for nursing. *Computers in Nursing* 7(5): 203–208.

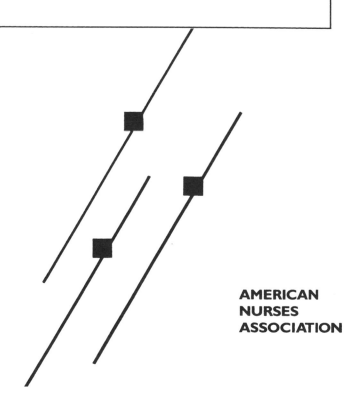

*Standards of
Practice for*

Nursing
Informatics

**AMERICAN
NURSES
ASSOCIATION**

STANDARDS of PRACTICE
for
Nursing
Informatics

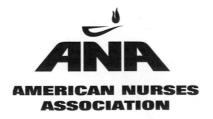

This document was developed by the American Nurses Association's Task Force to Develop Measurement Criteria for Standards for Nursing Informatics.

Task Force to Develop Measurement Criteria for Standards for Nursing Informatics

Susan D. McDermott, R.N., M.B.A.
Barbara Happ, Ph.D., R.N.
Judy A. Zimmet, R.N., C.N.M., M.S.N., M.S.I.S.
Judith S. Ronald, Ed.D., R.N.
Carole A. Gassert, Ph.D., R.N.
Linda L. Lange, Ed.D., R.N.
Diane Skiba, Ph.D. (NLN)
Mary McAlindon, Ed.D., R.N., C.N.A.A. (AMIA)
Patricia A. Abbott, M.S., R.N. (AMIA)
Lynda Joseph, R.N., M.S.N. (CHIM)
Cynthia Spurr, M.B.A., R.N. (HIMSS)

ANA Staff: D. Kathy Milholland, Ph.D., R.N., Senior Policy Fellow, Research and Databases, Department of Practice, Economics, and Policy

Published by
American Nurses Publishing
600 Maryland Avenue, SW
Suite 100 West
Washington, DC 20024-2571

CONTENTS

NURSING INFORMATICS
STANDARDS OF PRACTICE

This document sets forth standards of practice for the specialty of nursing informatics. Nursing informatics is the combination of nursing science, computer science, and information science. Standards are authoritative statements in which the nursing profession describes the responsibilities for which nurses are accountable. Consequently, standards reflect the values and priorities of the profession. Standards provide direction for professional nursing practice and a framework for the evaluation of practice. Standards are measurable criteria which define the nursing profession's accountability to the public and the outcomes for which nurses are responsible. Standards are relatively enduring while the criteria by which they are measured may change to reflect new knowledge and technology in current practice.

Nursing Informatics Standards of Practice describe a generalist level of practice and professional performance common to nurses engaged in nursing informatics practice. These standards apply to nurses who are qualified by experience and education to practice at the generalist level in nursing informatics.

The standards address nursing informatics practice provided to patients and clients. **Patient** refers to any person who is a direct recipient of clinical health services. **Client** is used in reference to all other recipients of the informatics nurse's practice. Other recipients include nurses, administrators, educators, researchers, healthcare practitioners, informatics professionals, other professional groups, and communities.

Nursing informatics focuses on the methods and tools of information handling in nursing practice. Nursing practice includes all areas of nursing endeavor, such as patient care, research, education, administration, and informatics. Information handling includes identifying, naming, organizing, grouping, collecting, processing, analyzing, storing, retrieving, communicating, transforming, or managing data or information.

PRACTICE STANDARDS FOR
THE INFORMATICS NURSE

Standard I. Assessment: Information Systems to Collect Patient and Client Data

THE INFORMATICS NURSE ANALYZES, DESIGNS, DEVELOPS, MODIFIES, IMPLEMENTS, EVALUATES, OR MAINTAINS INFORMATION HANDLING TECHNOLOGIES THAT COLLECT PATIENT AND CLIENT DATA TO SUPPORT THE PRACTICE OF NURSING.

Measurement Criteria

The informatics nurse:
1. Identifies data elements appropriate to a given practice context.
2. Identifies data needs using systems analysis techniques.
3. Analyzes workflow related to data collection in the target environment.
4. Analyzes, designs, develops, modifies, implements, evaluates, or maintains systems for efficient data collection.
5. Analyzes, designs, develops, modifies, implements, evaluates, or maintains information technologies to store collected data in a retrievable form.
6. Modifies information technologies to meet changing data requirements/needs.
7. Develops, implements, and evaluates procedures for achieving data integrity and security.
8. Supports efforts toward development and use of a unified nursing language.
9. Supports integration of a unified nursing language with the standardized language developed in collaboration with other health care disciplines.

10. Analyzes, designs, develops, modifies, implements, evaluates, or maintains information handling technologies that reflect nursing theories and models used in the practice setting.
11. Analyzes, designs, develops, modifies, implements, evaluates, or maintains information handling technologies that allow integration with policies, procedures, and knowledge bases related to collection of patient and client data.

Standard II. Diagnosis: Information Technologies That Utilize Patient and Client Data to Support Decision-making

THE INFORMATICS NURSE ANALYZES, DESIGNS, DEVELOPS, MODIFIES, IMPLEMENTS, EVALUATES, OR MAINTAINS INFORMATION HANDLING TECHNOLOGIES THAT USE PATIENT AND CLIENT DATA TO SUPPORT DECISION-MAKING.

Measurement Criteria

The informatics nurse:
1. Identifies the information required by the decision situation and the means to obtain it.
2. Analyzes, designs, develops, modifies, implements, evaluates, or maintains information handling technologies that provide decision support appropriate to the patient or the client.
3. Develops presentations of data that are useful for decision-making.
4. Analyzes, designs, develops, modifies, implements, evaluates, or maintains information handling technologies that aggregate, integrate, and transform data for decision-making.
5. Ensures that comprehensive, accurate, and timely data are available for decision-making.
6. Modifies information handling technologies to meet changing decision requirements.

7. Analyzes, designs, develops, modifies, implements, evaluates, or maintains information handling technologies that integrate policies, procedures, and knowledge bases related to decision-making.

Standard III. Identification of Outcomes: Information Handling Technologies That Provide for Identification of Outcomes for Patients and Clients

THE INFORMATICS NURSE ANALYZES, DESIGNS, DEVELOPS, MODIFIES, IMPLEMENTS, EVALUATES, OR MAINTAINS INFORMATION HANDLING TECHNOLOGIES THAT PROVIDE FOR IDENTIFICATION OF OUTCOMES FOR PATIENTS AND CLIENTS.

Measurement Criteria

The informatics nurse:
1. Collaborates with experts to identify measurable outcomes.
2. Analyzes, designs, develops, modifies, implements, evaluates, or maintains information handling technologies that support entry, retrieval, and analysis of identified outcomes.
3. Analyzes, designs, develops, modifies, implements, evaluates, or maintains systems that integrate and transform relevant data for identification of outcomes.
4. Analyzes, designs, develops, modifies, implements, evaluates, or maintains information handling technologies that include a time estimate for attainment of outcomes, that provide direction for continuity of care, that are suitable for analysis of aggregate data, and that are attainable with available resources.
5. Analyzes, designs, develops, modifies, implements, evaluates, or maintains information handling technologies that allow integration with policies, procedures, and knowledge bases related to identification of outcomes.

Standard IV. Planning: Information Handling Technologies to Develop Plans for Achieving Identified Outcomes

THE INFORMATICS NURSE ANALYZES, DESIGNS, DEVELOPS, MODIFIES, IMPLEMENTS, EVALUATES, OR MAINTAINS INFORMATION HANDLING TECHNOLOGIES TO DEVELOP PLANS FOR ACHIEVING IDENTIFIED OUTCOMES.

Measurement Criteria

The informatics nurse:
1. Analyzes, designs, develops, modifies, implements, evaluates, or maintains information handling technologies in which plans can be developed, modified, documented, and evaluated.
2. Analyzes, designs, develops, modifies, implements, evaluates, or maintains information handling technologies that support prioritization of activities within plans.
3. Supports information handling technologies that integrate and transform relevant data in the development of plans.
4. Analyzes, designs, develops, modifies, implements, evaluates, or maintains information handling technologies that present alternative plans for achieving identified outcomes.
5. Analyzes, designs, develops, modifies, implements, evaluates, or maintains information handling technologies that support interdisciplinary planning.
6. Analyzes, designs, develops, modifies, implements, evaluates, or maintains information handling technologies that integrate policies, procedures, and knowledge bases related to planning the achievement of identified outcomes.

Standard V. Implementation: Information Handling Technologies to Support Implementation of Plans

THE INFORMATICS NURSE ANALYZES, DESIGNS, DEVELOPS, MODIFIES, IMPLEMENTS, EVALUATES, OR MAINTAINS INFORMATION HANDLING TECHNOLOGIES TO DOCUMENT IMPLEMENTATION OF THE PLAN.

Measurement Criteria

The informatics nurse:
1. Analyzes, designs, develops, modifies, implements, evaluates, or maintains information handling technologies for documentation of activities and/or interventions.
2. Analyzes, designs, develops, modifies, implements, evaluates, or maintains information handling technologies that document and display planned activities and interventions to facilitate implementing the plan.
3. Supports information handling technologies that link documentation of interventions and/or activities to assessment data, decisions made, and outcomes identified.
4. Analyzes, designs, develops, modifies, implements, evaluates, or maintains information handling technologies that integrate policies, procedures, practice standards and clinical guidelines, and knowledge bases related to plan implementation.

Standard VI. Evaluation: Information Handling Technologies to Provide for Measurement and Evaluation of Outcomes

THE INFORMATICS NURSE ANALYZES, DESIGNS, DEVEL-OPS, MODIFIES, IMPLEMENTS, EVALUATES, OR MAIN-TAINS INFORMATION HANDLING TECHNOLOGIES TO PROVIDE FOR OUTCOME MEASUREMENT AND EVALUA-TION.

Measurement Criteria

The informatics nurse:
1. Analyzes, designs, develops, modifies, implements, evaluates, or maintains information handling technologies that allow data to be retrieved, aggregated, and made available for systematic and ongoing evaluation of outcomes.
2. Supports information handling technologies that allow evaluation of the effectiveness and efficiency of decisions, plans, and activities in relation to outcomes.
3. Analyzes, designs, develops, modifies, implements, evaluates, or maintains information handling technologies that identify variances and trends through analysis of outcomes and evaluations.
4. Analyzes, designs, develops, modifies, implements, evaluates, or maintains information handling technologies that use data from outcomes evaluation to develop or revise practice.

NURSING INFORMATICS STANDARDS OF PROFESSIONAL PERFORMANCE

Standard I. Quality of Nursing Informatics Practice

THE INFORMATICS NURSE SYSTEMATICALLY EVALU-
ATES THE QUALITY AND EFFECTIVENESS OF NURSING
INFORMATICS PRACTICE.

Measurement Criteria

The informatics nurse:
1. Identifies aspects of nursing informatics practice important for quality monitoring.
2. Identifies indicators used to monitor quality and effectiveness of nursing informatics practice.
3. Collects data to monitor quality and effectiveness of nursing informatics practice.
4. Analyzes quality data to identify opportunities for
   improving nursing informatics practice.
5. Formulates recommendations to improve nursing informatics practice or outcomes.
6. Implements activities to enhance the quality of nursing
   informatics practice.
7. Participates on interdisciplinary teams that evaluate nursing informatics practice or health informatics services.
8. Develops, implements, and evaluates policies and procedures to improve the quality of nursing informatics practice.
9. Recommends change in health care informatics using
   results from the evaluation of the quality and effectiveness
   of nursing informatics practice.

Standard II. Performance Appraisal

THE INFORMATICS NURSE EVALUATES OWN NURSING PRACTICE IN RELATION TO PROFESSIONAL PRACTICE STANDARDS AND RELEVANT STATUTES AND REGULATIONS.

Measurement Criteria

The informatics nurse:
1. Engages in performance appraisal on a regular basis, identifying areas of strength as well as areas for professional/practice development.
2. Seeks constructive feedback regarding own practice.
3. Takes action to achieve goals identified during performance appraisal.
4. Participates in peer review as appropriate.
5. Complies with professional standards and regulations.
6. Develops performance appraisal procedures related to nursing informatics practice.

Standard III. Education

THE INFORMATICS NURSE ACQUIRES AND MAINTAINS CURRENT KNOWLEDGE IN NURSING INFORMATICS PRACTICE.

Measurement Criteria

The informatics nurse:
1. Seeks additional knowledge and skills appropriate to the practice setting by participating in educational programs and activities, conferences, workshops, interdisciplinary professional meetings, and self-directed learning.
2. Keeps a record of own learning activities.
3. Seeks certification when eligible.

Standard IV. Collegiality

**THE INFORMATICS NURSE CONTRIBUTES TO THE PRO-
FESSIONAL DEVELOPMENT OF PEERS, COLLEAGUES,
AND OTHERS.**

Measurement Criteria

The informatics nurse:
1. Shares knowledge and skills.
2. Contributes to informatics education of students, peers, and colleagues.
3. Provides constructive feedback regarding others' practice.
4. Promotes understanding and effective use of information technology.
5. Promotes understanding of nursing informatics.

Standard V. Ethics

**THE INFORMATICS NURSE'S DECISIONS AND ACTIONS
ON BEHALF OF PATIENTS AND CLIENTS ARE BASED ON
ETHICAL PRINCIPLES.**

Measurement Criteria

The informatics nurse:
1. Practices according to the Code for Nurses.[1]
2. Maintains privacy, confidentiality, and security of patient and client data.
3. Acts as an advocate of system users, both patients and clients.
4. Practices in a nonjudgmental and nondiscriminatory manner that is sensitive to human diversity.
5. Practices in a manner that preserves and protects human autonomy, dignity, and rights.
6. Seeks available resources to help formulate ethical decisions.
7. Protects patient and client data from unauthorized use.

8. Incorporates relevant laws and regulations into informatics practice.

Standard VI. Collaboration

THE INFORMATICS NURSE COLLABORATES WITH OTHERS IN THE CONDUCT OF NURSING INFORMATICS PRACTICE.

Measurement Criteria

The informatics nurse:
1. Collaborates with patients and clients.
2. Makes referrals and recommendations as needed.
3. Collaborates with other disciplines in teaching, consultation, management, research, and system development.
4. Collaborates with informatics nurses, informatics nurse specialists, and other nurses.

Standard VII. Research

THE INFORMATICS NURSE CONTRIBUTES TO THE BODY OF INFORMATICS KNOWLEDGE.

Measurement Criteria

The informatics nurse:
1. Identifies problems suitable for nursing informatics research.
2. Participates in research activities.
3. Serves on research committees.
4. Applies appropriate research to nursing informatics practice.
5. Participates in research dissemination activities.
6. Develops policies, procedures, and guidelines based on research.

Standard VIII. Resource Utilization

**THE INFORMATICS NURSE CONSIDERS FACTORS RELAT-
ED TO SAFETY, EFFECTIVENESS, COST, AND SOCIAL
IMPACT IN CONDUCTING INFORMATICS PRACTICE.**

Measurement Criteria

The informatics nurse:
1. Evaluates factors related to safety, effectiveness, cost, and social impact when developing and implementing information handling technologies.
2. Assigns tasks or delegates responsibilities appropriately based on the nursing informatics activity being conducted.

DOMAIN STANDARDS FOR
THE INFORMATICS NURSE

Standard I. Information System Life Cycle

THE INFORMATICS NURSE APPLIES KNOWLEDGE AND SKILLS OF THE INFORMATION SYSTEMS LIFE CYCLE TO PRACTICE.

Measurement Criteria

The informatics nurse:
1. Conducts systems analysis.
2. Identifies information handling technology requirements for nursing practice.
3. Analyzes, designs, develops, modifies, implements, evaluates, or maintains information handling technologies for nursing practice.
4. Analyzes, designs, develops, modifies, implements, evaluates, or maintains information systems using software tools.
5. Selects information handling technologies for nursing practice.
6. Conducts tests of information handling technologies.
7. Conducts educational programs for clients and patients.
8. Implements information handling technologies.
9. Evaluates information handling technologies' performance and impact on nursing practice.
10. Recommends information handling technologies and nursing practice enhancements using information handling technologies evaluation data.
11. Maintains information handling technologies through updating and modifying components to meet changing nursing practice requirements.

12. Conducts feasibility assessments throughout the information systems life cycle.
13. Documents activities related to information systems life cycle.
14. Directs or participates in efforts to continuously upgrade the quality and effectiveness of information handling technologies.
15. Develops policies and procedures related to information systems implementations.
16. Analyzes, designs, develops, modifies, implements, evaluates, or maintains information handling technologies that adhere to established law.

Standard II. Principles and Theory

THE INFORMATICS NURSE APPLIES KNOWLEDGE AND PRINCIPLES FROM NURSING AND SUPPORTING DISCIPLINES TO PRACTICE.

Supporting disciplines include computer science, information science, behavioral science, management science, cognitive science, communication theory, telecommunications, education, mathematics, and engineering.

Measurement Criteria

The informatics nurse:
1. Applies knowledge from classical and current literature to direct nursing informatics practice.
2. Synthesizes principles and theories from nursing and supporting disciplines to direct nursing informatics practice.

Standard III. Information Technology

THE INFORMATICS NURSE IS PROFICIENT IN THE APPLICATION OF INFORMATION HANDLING TECHNOLOGIES.

Examples of information handling technologies include, but are not limited to computers, telecommunications, networks, physiological monitors, imaging devices, interfaces, scanners, printers, architecture, and software.

Measurement Criteria

The informatics nurse:
1. Applies new information handling technologies to practice.
2. Optimizes opportunities for applying information handling technologies to nursing practice.
3. Employs technology assessment methods in evaluating information handling technologies.
4. Explains information handling technologies in a way that allows clients to be informed consumers.
5. Teaches clients about effective and ethical uses of information handling technologies in nursing practice.
6. Applies ergonomic principles in the selection and use of information handling technologies.

Standard IV. Communication

THE INFORMATICS NURSE COMMUNICATES WITH CLIENTS, SUPPORTING DISCIPLINES, AND OTHERS IN HEALTHCARE ORGANIZATIONS.

Measurement Criteria

The informatics nurse:
1. Is fluent in informatics and nursing terminologies.
2. Articulates client needs and requirements to other disciplines.
3. Interprets information handling technologies-related information from other disciplines for clients and patients.
4. Interprets communications from other disciplines to clients and patients.

Standard V. Databases

THE INFORMATICS NURSE ANALYZES, DESIGNS, DEVEL-
OPS, MODIFIES, IMPLEMENTS, EVALUATES, OR MAINTAINS
STRUCTURES FOR ORGANIZING, STORING, EDITING,
RETRIEVING, AND ANALYZING DATA THAT SUPPORT
THE PRACTICE OF NURSING.

Measurement Criteria

The informatics nurse:
1. Integrates nursing taxonomies, unified nomenclatures, and other data needed by nurses within database design.
2. Incorporates established data and database management standards into database design.
3. Assists clients in using databases to make data-driven decisions.
4. Develops procedures to establish and maintain the validity and integrity of data and databases.
5. Promotes the integrity of nursing information and access necessary for patient care within an integrated computer-based patient record.
6. Supports the development of integrated computer-based patient record technologies.

Reference

1. Code for Nurses with Interpretive Statements. Kansas City, MO: American Nurses Association; 1985.

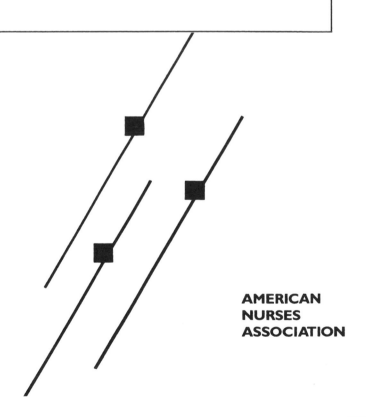

Scope of
Practice for Nursing Informatics

**AMERICAN
NURSES
ASSOCIATION**

This document was developed by the American Nurses Association's Task Force on the Scope of Practice for Nursing Informatics.

Task Force on the Scope of Practice for Nursing Informatics

Mary L. McHugh, Ph.D., R.N., A.R.N.P.
Patricia Flatley Brennan, Ph.D., R.N.
Bennie Harsanyi, Ph.D., R.N.
Susan McDermott, M.S., R.N.
Judy Ozbolt, Ph.D., R.N.
Roy Simpson, R.N., C., F.N.A.P.
Diane Skiba, Ph.D.

ANA Staff: D. Kathy Milholland, Ph.D., R.N., Senior Policy Fellow, Research and Databases, Department of Practice, Economics, and Policy

Published by
American Nurses Publishing
600 Maryland Avenue, SW
Suite 100 West
Washington, DC 20024-2571

Definition and Terms

As a scientific discipline, nursing informatics serves the profession of nursing by supporting the information handling work of other nursing specialties. Nursing informatics is the specialty that integrates nursing science, computer science, and information science in identifying, collecting, processing, and managing data and information to support nursing practice, administration, education, research, and the expansion of nursing knowledge. It supports the practice of all nursing specialties, in all sites and settings of care, whether at the basic or advanced practice level.

The practice of nursing informatics includes the development and evaluation of applications, tools, processes, and structures which assist nurses with the management of data in taking care of patients or in supporting the practice of nursing. It includes adapting or customizing existing informatics technology to the requirements of nurses. It involves collaboration with other health care and informatics professionals in the development of informatics products and standards for nursing and health care informatics.

Though competence in the use of applications software is a prerequisite for nursing informatics practice, it is insufficient to define that practice. Nurses who practice in the field of nursing informatics are designated, "informatics nurses." This term is preferred because it is consistent with nursing terminology for other areas of practice (e.g., psychiatric nurse). It recognizes that the person is *both* a nurse and an informaticist.

The term, informatics, denotes the activities involved in identifying, naming, organizing, grouping, collecting, processing, analyzing, storing, retrieving, or managing data and information. The term, *information handling*, defines all the informatics activities of nurses. The term, *nursing practice*, includes all areas of nursing endeavor—e.g., patient care, research, education, administration, and informatics.

The terms, *patient* and *client* differentiate between two sets of recipients of the services of informatics nurses. *Patient* refers to any person who is in the system as a direct recipient of clinical health care services. *Client* refers to all other recipients of the informatics nurse's services.

Boundaries

This section discusses both what nursing informatics is, and what it is not. Nursing informatics practice encompasses the full range of activities that focus on information handling in nursing. Nursing informatics is a support function that serves to assist all nurses in doing the work of nursing in an efficient and effective manner. All nurses perform some information handling activities. Yet, not all nurses are informaticists.

The core product of nursing is patient care. In support of patient care, nursing practice expanded to nursing research, education, and administration, and, more recently, informatics. The support technologies of nursing research, education, and administration exist to support the highest possible quality patient care, as does nursing informatics. It may do this directly by supporting nurses engaged in clinical patient care, or indirectly by supporting nursing education, research, and administration. Thus, nursing informatics extends its support and influence into all other areas of nursing practice.

Nursing Informatics Distinguished from Other Areas of Nursing Practice

Nursing informatics is distinguished from other nursing specialties by its special focus on the information of nursing, i.e., the methods and technology of information handling in nursing. The particular substance of the information is not the primary focus of nursing informatics. Other nursing specialties focus on the substance of the information with which they are concerned; they use informatics methods and tools to advance their understanding of the content of the nursing information. It is the melding of nursing knowledge with non-nursing knowledge bases related to informatics that constitutes nursing informatics practice.

The content and context of the substance of the information are not unimportant to the informatics nurse. The reason informatics *nurses* are needed is that specialized nursing knowledge requires handling that is consistent with the requirements of the nurse users. Nurses are best able to describe and define the requirements of nurse users.

Nursing Informatics Spans Clinical and Non-Clinical Practice

Nursing informatics is a practice discipline. The informatics nurse may or may not be in clinical practice. The determination is found in the proximity of the product to patient care. Whenever the work of informatics nurses concentrates on the handling of patient care information, the informatics nurse is functioning in the clinical domain. When the work of the informatics nurse targets nursing education, research, administration, or pure informatics, the nurse may or may not be functioning in the clinical domain. In many cases, the work of the informatics nurse is designed to serve patients directly. Competent nursing practice is dependent on the availability of complete and accurate information about patients' health care needs and nursing care requirements. To the extent that the informatics nurse focuses on direct provision of information to the patient care process, the informatics nurse is functioning in the clinical domain.

Nursing Informatics Distinguished from Other Informatics Disciplines

The boundaries of nursing informatics overlap those of other scientific disciplines and domains such as mathematics, statistics, engineering, and computer science. These areas of overlap involve the development and application of algorithms and structures used for handling, communicating, and transforming data into knowledge and new discoveries. The boundaries of these fields are not rigid: they are dynamic, fluid, and rapidly expanding, allowing for exchange of information and adapting to changes in the internal and external environment.

Systems Integration and the Informatics Nurse

One boundary issue must be clearly addressed in the scope of nursing informatics practice—the positioning of nursing informatics within the larger arena of health informatics. Nurses function as members of health care teams. The information systems used by health care teams must adequately serve the requirements of all members of the team. This requirement is best met with *integrated systems*.

The services of informatics nurses are required if the integrated systems are to serve patients and health professionals successfully by assuring that the nursing perspective is available in such systems. It is the responsibility of the informatics nurse to protect the integrity of nursing information and nurses' access to information necessary for patient care within an integrated, computer-based patient record.

Research has shown that complex systems are more likely to fail when end-users are not consulted during the design phase. To achieve high-quality performance, integrated systems must be designed so the needs of each category of user are considered at *all* phases of information systems development and implementation.

Informatics nurses work within the context of collaborative systems-design teams. Though their unique responsibility is to ensure that the integrated health-care information systems adequately meet nursing information needs, this does not mean nursing systems are to be separate from systems used by other members of the health care team.

Core

The *core phenomena* of nursing informatics are all data, information, and knowledge involved in nursing. The *core operations* of nursing informatics are identifying, acquiring, preserving, managing, retrieving, aggregating, analyzing, and transmitting this data, information, and knowledge to make it meaningful and useful to nurses. The technology that facilitates these operations is, of course, also of concern to nursing informatics.

Because nursing is information-intensive as well as information-dependent, the theory and practice of nursing informatics are fundamental to the discipline and the profession. At the most basic level—the symbolic representation of nursing phenomena—nursing informatics concerns include but are not limited to:

- Terminology (naming conventions for nursing phenomena)
- Classifications and taxonomies
- Graphic, visual, and audio depictions of nursing phenomena
- Procedural and algorithmic representations of nursing phenomena.

Nursing informatics theory addresses the ways nurses use data, information, and knowledge to make decisions and deliver care. In addition, it is concerned with the technologies for information management and processing and how these modalities affect and are affected by the practice of nursing.

Instances of Nursing Informatics Practice

Nursing informatics practice has the following characteristics:

- The content of the information is related to nursing;
- The technology is designed to facilitate some aspect of information handling, communication, or transformation.
- The technology itself is an information handling, communication, or transformation technology.
- The technology is used in such a way that nursing information is handled, communicated, or transformed. And,
- The focus of the activity is information handling, communication, or transformation rather than patient care or education, research, or administration.

The development and application of information-handling methods and tools related to nursing practice is informatics, regardless of the setting in which nursing is practiced. Writing a spreadsheet program to support nursing care of patients is an example of the practice of nursing informatics. Use of nursing informatics knowledge to improve quality of nursing care by helping nurse managers develop systems for the effective use of nursing resources is an instance of nursing informatics practice.

Daily use of a word processor by the nurse giving care to patients is not, by itself, an instance of nursing informatics practice. Use of a computerized patient-classification system is not, by itself, informatics practice.

The following are additional examples of nursing informatics practice: developing a naming system and/or a related taxonomy to describe and order nursing phenomena; computerizing a manual nursing-record document or system; designing or developing a computer program for an interactive video disc system; developing methods for documenting nursing information in either a paper- or computer-based record system; setting up computer program applications to be used by nurses in clinical practice; or developing or testing new theory pertaining to handling, communicating, or transforming nursing information.

The following activities would not, *by themselves*, constitute instances of nursing informatics practice: use of a word processor to teach students about nursing or word processors; use of a spreadsheet in the conduct of clinical research; teaching a course in computers in nursing; use of the data in a computer-based patient record to manage nursing care; or use of the data in a database management system to manage a nursing service.

Intersections with Other Disciplines

Nursing informatics is one element of the broader field of health informatics, an amalgam of health and information sciences. Nursing informatics intersects with the disciplines and domains concerned with the conceptual, cognitive, and mechanical structures and algorithms used to manage data, information, and knowledge. These intersections or overlaps contribute to the delivery of professional nursing care, the generation of nursing knowledge, and the achievement of health for individuals, families, and communities.

This statement of the scope of nursing informatics does not limit the boundary or fix the intersections of nursing informatics with other professions. Instead, it allows for expansion based on the reality of constant change in nursing, in all of health care, and in technology.

Nursing informatics is concerned with two kinds of intersections—one with supporting disciplines and one with collaborating health and related service providers. Supporting disciplines can be subsumed under the term, informatics, and include such diverse areas as computer science, psychology, management information science, organizational science, engineering, library science, information management, communication theory, and decision sciences.

The intersections are dynamic in nature and variable across time. They are driven by changes within and outside nursing. Important areas where changes within nursing can influence the nature and type of intersections include: changing roles of nurses, nursing science, and demands for nursing research. Changes from outside the discipline will also alter the nature of intersections needed. Examples of areas where these changes can occur include: technology, finance, economics, management science, health care delivery systems, and public policy.

All health care professions interact, share the same overall mission, have access to the same published scientific knowledge, and, to some degree, overlap. In the practice setting, nursing informatics applications do not exist alone. Nursing uses programs and data sets common to many clinical disciplines. Nursing informatics assumes an important role in ensuring that nursing's data and knowledge are structured in such a way that they are accepted and accessible to the larger health care community. Because nursing utilizes information for purposes different from those of other clinical disciplines, it may require programs and information management tools that are tailored to the unique goals of clinical nursing.

The informatics nurse needs to have a vision of the intersections necessary to support practice in a restructured health care system with its focus on consumers, and with services encompassing traditional care facilities as well as diverse community-based facilities in locations such as schools and workplaces.

Dimensions of Nursing Informatics

Statement of Beliefs

1. Nursing informatics ultimately serves the interests of patients.
2. Nursing informatics is intrinsic to nursing care.
3. Nursing informatics facilitates the efforts of nurses and nursing to improve the quality of nursing care and the welfare of patients.
4. Nursing informatics serves to assure the quality and cost-effectiveness of care by providing nurse clinicians with data,

information, and knowledge necessary to assess the cost and efficacy of nursing care.

5. Nursing informatics facilitates health-care effectiveness research by aggregating clinical data and making these data amenable to analysis.

6. Nursing informatics is responsible for the protection of the confidentiality and privacy of personal health information.

7. Nursing informatics is responsible for promoting safe patient care by developing systems that help evaluate the quality of nursing care.

8. Nursing informatics promotes the use of technology to monitor nursing practices and associated patient outcomes in the following ways:

   a. developing systems to determine the statistical limits of acceptable nursing care outcomes;

   b. structuring these systems so as to promote patient welfare and fairness simultaneously to nurses whose practice is monitored;

   c. developing systems that can be used by nurses to identify and specify the boundaries of nursing-mediated patient outcomes;

   d. identifying nursing practices that lie outside those boundaries (i.e., that have unusual success or failure rates); and,

   e. furthering the science of nursing by making that information available to the profession.

9. Nursing information systems are designed to serve nurses rather than to be served by nurses.

10. Nursing informatics promotes design and development of valid and reliable decision-support systems and facilitates their availability.

11. Nursing informatics contributes to the body of knowledge of health care informatics.

12. Advanced practice in nursing informatics requires preparation at the graduate level in nursing.

Roles of Informatics Nurses

The work of an informatics nurse can involve any and all phases of the life cycle of nursing information systems: theory formulation, design, development, marketing, selection, testing, implementation, training, use, maintenance, evaluation, and enhancement.

Informatics nurses are needed to:

- develop theory and methods of inquiry in nursing informatics.
- develop or collaborate in the development of manual and computer information systems.
- conduct the research that underlies the design and development of information systems. This includes:
  a. basic research on symbolic representation of nursing phenomena.
  b. basic research on clinical decision making in nursing.
  c. applied research and development of prototype systems.
  d. ergonomic research on the effects of systems on nurses, patients, and nursing care.
  e. evaluation research on the effects of systems on the processes and outcomes of nursing care.
- Conduct research using data aggregated and made available by nursing and other information systems. For example:
  a. verifying the Nursing Minimum Data Set with clinical records.
  b. mapping nursing notes on to controlled vocabularies.
- Teach nurses, nursing students, and others about the effective and ethical uses of information technology in nursing practice.
- Participate in the process of making quality information systems available and useable to nurses.

Human Resource Considerations

Minimum Informatics Competencies for the Profession

There are a set of competencies needed by all nurses, regardless of practice level or setting. Nursing informatics is distinguished from other specialties by its concern with the symbolic representation of nursing information and systems for dealing with that information.

The most fundamental informatics requirements for all practitioners involve identifying information requirements for practice, documenting care, and protecting the confidentiality and privacy of patient information. Nurses must access information resources needed for clinical practice. Finally, a basic expectation is that all nurses demonstrate minimum competence in the use of available information technologies required to provide nursing care in their practice settings.

The following competencies are required for graduates of basic nursing programs:

- identify, collect, and record data relevant to the nursing care of patients;
- analyze and interpret patient and nursing information as part of the planning for and provision of nursing services;
- employ health-care informatics applications designed for the clinical practice of nursing; and,
- implement public and institutional policies related to privacy, confidentiality, and security of information. These include patient care information, confidential employer information, and other information gained in the nurse's professional capacity.

Preparation for Practice in Nursing Informatics

Nursing Informatics Practice

An informatics nurse has a bachelor's degree in nursing and additional knowledge and experience in the field of informatics. Requisite competencies for nursing informatics practice include:

- Systems analysis.
- Systems design.
- Development of structures for organizing data and databases.
- Testing and evaluating applications for nursing.
- Consultation on the configuration of hardware and software to meet nursing's needs.
- Knowledge about the workings of computers and how computer information resources need to function to support nursing practice.
- The technologies, methodologies, and processes involved in the interface between nurses and information technologies used to support nursing practice.
- Bi-cultural and bilingual skills sufficient to serve as a translator between nurses and the engineers, analysts, and system designers who develop and implement information systems designed to support nursing practice.
- Use of applications software.
- Networks and distributed information resources.
- Employment of computer programming tools and utilities in the accomplishment of nursing informatics work.
- Employment of principles from supporting disciplines as needed.

Additional skills valuable in the practice of nursing informatics are:

- Competence in the development of hardware and software necessary for the practice of nursing informatics.
- Functional skill in hardware (e.g., installation, setup, and maintenance of computer hardware/components).
- Software installation and maintenance (original installation, debugging, and updating).

- Writing software in one or more computer languages—e.g., C, Cobol, Fortran, or Basic.
- Skills in integrating two or more computer systems.
- Ability to coordinate projects of various sizes involving diverse team members and constituencies.

Specialist Practice in Nursing Informatics

An *informatics nurse specialist* (INS) has a master's degree in nursing and has taken graduate-level courses in the field of informatics. The INS is prepared to assume roles requiring advanced knowledge in nursing and in informatics.

Specialists in nursing informatics must be competent in the following areas:

- The design and/or implementation of applications of nursing informatics science to nursing practice problems.
- Analysis and evaluation of information requirements for nursing practice.
- Appraisal of computer and information technologies for their applicability to nursing practice problems. This includes:
  a. appraisal of the appropriateness of the technology to the nursing situation,
  b. appraisal of the effectiveness of the proposed technology to the specific problem,
  c. appraisal of the impact of the proposed technology on nursing efficiency and productivity, and
  d. analysis of any ethical issues pertaining to proposed applications of information technology to nursing practice—especially those concerned with patient safety and privacy.
- Developing and teaching theory and practice of nursing informatics.
- Consultation practice in the field of nursing informatics. Consultation clients may include (but are not limited to) administrators, nurse practitioners, nurse educators, nurse researchers, vendors of information technology with health care applications, and other consulting firms.

- Collaboration with other health informatics specialists and other specialists from supporting disciplines in the creation or application of informatics theory and practice for nurses and/or nursing.
- Development of strategies, policies, and procedures for introducing, evaluating, and modifying information technology applied to nursing practice.

INDEX

An index entry preceded by a bracketed calendar year indicates an entry from a previous edition or predecessor publication that is included in this edition as an appendix. Thus: [2001] is *Scope and Standards of Nursing Informatics Practice* (Appendix A).; [1995] is *Standards of Practice for Nursing Informatics* (Appendix B); [1994] is *Scope of Practice for Nursing Informatics* (Appendix C).

A

Access to health information, 26, 43, 44
  advocacy for, 87
  balance of privacy and, 21, 47–48
    passim, 52, 56–62 *passim*
Access to health services, 6, 22, 27
Accountability, 79, 87
Administration, leadership, and
    management (NI functional area),
    18–19
Advanced practice in NI. *See*
    Informatics Nurse Specialist (INS)
Advocacy, 24, 47, 87–88
  coordination of activities and, 72
  ethics and, 83
  [2001], 142
  [1995], 167
  resource utilization and
  [2001], 144
  standard of professional performance,
    87–88
  for user access and security, 48–49
American Medical Informatics
    Association (AMIA), 40
American Nurses Association (ANA)
  code of ethics, 47, 83, 142, 167
  informatics activities of, 1–2, 7–9, 30,
    115–116
  See also Code of Ethics for Nurses
    with Interpretive Statements,
American Nurses Credentialing Center
    (ANCC), 17, 36
AMIA. *See* American Medical
    Informatics Association
Analysis
  as NI functional area, 19–20

of outcomes, 20
  See also Critical thinking, analysis, and
    synthesis
Assessment
  evaluation and, 76
  implementation and [1995], 163
  problem and issues identification, 68
    [2001], 133–134
  standard of practice, 67
    [1995], 159–160
  as step in nursing process, 65
    [2001], 132

B

Bioinformatics. *See* Health informatics
Body of knowledge, 46,
  assessment and [1995], 160
  collaboration and [2001], 143
  databases and [1995], 173
  education and, 77
    [1995], 166
  implementation and [1995], 163
  outcomes identification and [1995], 161
  planning and [1995], 162
  principles and theory [1995], 171
  quality of practice and, 79
  research and, 85
    [2001], 143
    [1995], 168
  See also Evidence-based practice

C

Care delivery models, 59–60
Care recipient. *See* Patient
Case management. *See* Coordination of
    activities

Data collection (*continued*)
quality of practice and, 79
[2001], 140
[1995], 165
research and, 85
Data element sets (ANA-recognized),
7–9
Decision-making and NI practice, 11–13,
20, 27, 28, 45, 54, 56, 65
[2001], 110–111, 132
advocacy and, 88
collaboration and, 82
databases and,
[1995], 173
diagnosis and,
[1995], 160–161
ethics and, 47–48, 84
[2001], 142
evaluation and,
[1995], 164
implementation and,
[1995], 163
leadership and, 90
planning and, 70
professional practice evaluation and,
78
research and, 85
Decision support systems (DSS), 12–13,
91
Development (NI functional area), 24–25
Devices and hardware and NI, 51–53
Diagnosis in NI practice
as step in nursing process, 65
[2001], 132
standard of practice,
[1995], 160–161
See also Problem and issues
identification
Distance learning, 26
Documentation and NI practice, 6, 9,
12, 19, 24, 29
assessment and, 67
collaboration and, 82
coordination of activities and, 72
databases and [1995], 173
education and, 77
[1995], 166

evaluation and, 76
[2001], 138, 139
implementation and, 71
[1995], 163
information systems life cycle and, 18
[1995], 171
outcomes identification and, 69
[2001], 135
planning and,
[2001], 136
[1995], 162
problem and issues identification, 68
quality of practice and, 79
Domain standards for NI [1995], 170–173
communication, 172
databases, 173
information system life cycle, 170
information technology, 171–172
principles and theory, 171
Domains of nursing practice, 20, 35
Domains of NI practice, 35–36, 43

E

Economic issues. *See* Cost control
Education of NI nurses, 25–27, 65
[2001], 104–105
[1994], 187–88
collaboration and, 82
[2001], 143
[1995], 168
collegiality and, 81
[2001], 142
[1995], 167
competencies and, 34–35
curricular design, 56, 58
evaluation and,
[2001], 139
as functional area of NI, 25–27
implementation and,
[2001], 137–138
information systems life cycle and, 18
[1995], 170
research and, 85
standard of professional performance,
77
[2001], 141
[1995], 166

technology trends in, 55–56
See also Mentoring; Professional development
Education of patients and families, 11, 12, 65, 74
  advocacy and, 87, 88
  assessment and, 67
  evaluation and, 76
  outcomes identification and, 69
  planning and, 70
  problem and issues identification, 68
  See also Family; Health teaching and health promotion; Patient
Education and professional development (NI functional area), 25–27
Educational technologies trends, 55–56
Electronic health records (EHRs). *See* Health records and records management
Environment of NI practice. *See* Practice environment
Ergonomics and usability, 10–11, 66, 133
  information technology and, [1995], 172
Ethics and NI, 47–48, 66, 133
  compliance and integrity management, 17, 21–22
  confidentiality, 21–22, 43, 47–48 *passim*, 52, 56– 62 *passim*, 83, 87, 137
  data integrity, security, and confidentiality, 21–22
  genomics, 21, 58
  healthcare informatics code (per IMIA), 47–48, 49
  implementation and, [2001], 137
  information technology and, [1995], 172
  quality of practice and, 79
  standard of professional performance, 83–84
  [2001], 142–143
  [1995], 167–168

See also Code of Ethics for Nurses with Interpretive Statements; Confidentiality and privacy
Evaluation in NI practice
  as functional area of NI, 28–29
  information system life cycle and, 18
  [1995], 170
  information technology and
  [1995], 172
  standard of practice, 76
  [2001], 138–139
  [1995], 164
  as step in nursing process, 65
  [2001], 132
Evidence-based practice
  assessment and, 67
  consultation and, 75
  education and, 77
  evaluation and, 76
  health teaching and health promotion, 73
  implementation and, 71
  outcomes identification and, 69
  quality of practice and, 80
  See also Research
Expert systems, 12, 13, 91
  See also Decision support systems

F
Family
  advocacy and, 87, 88
  assessment and, 67
  collaboration and, [2001], 143
  evaluation and, 76
  [2001], 138
  health teaching and health promotion, 74
  outcomes identification and, 69
  planning and, 70
  problem and issues identification, 68
  See also Education of patients and families; Patient
Financial issues. *See* Cost control
Functional areas for NI practice, 16–32
  administration, leadership, and management , 18–19

Internet, 74, 47–48, 49

J

Job titles and activities in NI, 16
  See also Functional areas for NI practice
Joint Commission on Accreditation of
    Healthcare Organizations (JCAHO),
    59, 60

K

Knowledge and NI practice, 65
  [2001], 105–108, 132
  as NI metastructure, 3–5, 12–13, 34
  representation trends, 54
  as synthesis of data and information,
    3, 4, 19, 45, 46, 54
  See also Metastructures . . . in NI;
    Wisdom and NI practice
Knowledge base. *See* Body of knowledge
Knowledge discovery in databases
    (KDDB), 19–20, 56

L

Laws, statutes, and regulations, 66
  [2001], 133
  ethics and, 83
    [1995], 168
  information systems life cycle and, 18
    [1995], 171
  planning and, 70
  problem and issues identification, 68
    [2001], 134
  professional practice evaluation and,
    78
    [2001], 141
    [1995], 166
  quality of practice and,
    [2001], 140
  standards and regulatory
    requirements, 24–25
  See also Ethics
Leadership,
  coordination of activities and, 72
  as functional area in NI, 18–19
  standard of professional
    performance, 89–90
  See also Mentoring

Licensing. *See* Certification and
    credentialing

M

Management as functional area in NI,
    18–19
Medical informatics. *See* AMIA; Health
    informatics; IMIA
Measurement criteria for NI practice, 67–90
  [2001], 133–145
  [1995], 159–173
  advocacy, 87–88
  assessment, 67
    [1995], 159–160
  collaboration, 82
    [2001], 143
    [1995], 168
  collegiality, 81
    [2001], 141–142
    [1995], 167
  communication,
    [2001], 144–145
  consultation, 75
  coordination of activities, 72
  diagnosis,
    [1995], 160–161
  education, 77
    [2001], 141
    [1995], 166
  ethics, 83–84
    [2001], 142–143
    [1995], 167–168
  evaluation, 76
    [2001], 138–139
    [1995], 164
  health teaching and health promotion,
    73–74
  implementation, 71
    [2001], 136–138
    [1995], 163
  leadership, 89–90
  outcomes identification, 69
    [2001], 134–135
    [1995], 161
  planning, 70
    [2001], 135–136
    [1995], 162